When Life Ends

When Life Ends

LEGAL OVERVIEWS, MEDICOLEGAL FORMS, AND HOSPITAL POLICIES

Arthur S. Berger

Foreword by Louis Lemberg

PRAEGER

Westport, Connecticut
London

Library of Congress Cataloging-in-Publication Data

Berger, Arthur S.
    When life ends : legal overviews, medicolegal forms, and hospital
policies / Arthur S. Berger ; foreword by Louis Lemberg.
      p.   cm.
    Includes bibliographical references and index.
    ISBN 0-275-94620-7 (alk. paper)
    1. Terminal care. 2. Terminal care—Law and legislation—United
States. 3. Terminally ill—Hospital care. 4. Do-not-resuscitate
orders. 5. Right to die. I. Title.
    [DNLM: 1. Right to Die—United States—legislation. 2. Advance
Directives—United States—legislation. 3. Terminal Care—United
States—legislation. 4. Hospital Administration—United States—
legislation. 5. Decision Making—United States—legislation.
6. Informed Consent—United States—legislation. W 32.5 AA1 B4w
1995]
R726.8.B467   1995
362.1'75—dc20
DNLM/DLC
for Library of Congress   94-43173

British Library Cataloguing in Publication Data is available.

Library of Congress Catalog Card Number: 94-43173
ISBN: 0-275-94620-7

First published in 1995

Praeger Publishers, 88 Post Road West, Westport, CT 06881
An imprint of Greenwood Publishing Group, Inc.

Printed in the United States of America

The paper used in this book complies with the
Permanent Paper Standard issued by the National
Information Standards Organization (Z39.48–1984).

10 9 8 7 6 5 4 3 2

Contents

Foreword by Louis Lemberg, M.D., Professor of Clinical Cardiology,
University of Miami School of Medicine   xi

Preface   xiii

Introduction   1

I   Legal Overviews   9

  1   Refusal of Life-Sustaining Treatment   11

    1.1 Right to Refuse Life-Sustaining Treatment   11

    1.2 Right of Refusal and State Interests   19

    1.3 Hospital Policy and Procedures—Refusal of Treatment by Patients
with Decision-Making Capacity and Without Decision-Making Capacity   23

    1.4 Limitation of Right of Refusal of Life-Sustaining Treatment to
Terminally Ill Patients   25

    1.5 Dependence of Right of Refusal on Whether Care Is Extraordinary
or Ordinary   25

    1.6 Termination of Life-Sustaining Treatment Already Begun   26

    1.7 Right of Refusal of Life-Sustaining Treatment and Artificial Feeding   26

    1.8 Right of Refusal of Medical Treatment and Euthanasia   27

    1.9 Right of Refusal and Institutional Policies   28

    1.10 Forcing Health Providers to Comply with Patients' Wishes   29

1.11 Termination of Life Support and Court Approval   30

2   Living Wills   33

2.1 Advance Directives   33

2.2 Living Will Statutes: Common Provisions   33

2.3 Living Wills: Form, Content, and Procedures   35

3   Surrogate Decision Making   43

3.1 Decision-Making Capacity and the Right to Refuse Treatment   43

3.2 Mechanisms for Health Care Decision Making: Health Care
Surrogate, Durable Power of Attorney for Health Care, and Proxy   45

3.3 Hospital Policy and Procedures—Patients with Advance Directives   52

3.4 Standards for Surrogate Decision Making   52

4   Termination of Treatment   55

4.1 Withholding or Withdrawing Life-Sustaining Treatment   55

4.2 Hospital Policies and Procedures—Withholding or Withdrawing
Life-Sustaining Treatment from Terminally Ill Adult and Pediatric
Patients   56

5   Withholding Cardiopulmonary Resuscitation   63

5.1 Do-Not-Resuscitate Order   63

5.2 Hospital Policy and Procedures—Do-Not-Resuscitate Order   69

5.3 Prehospital Do-Not-Resuscitate Order   73

6   Autonomy and the Federal Government   75

6.1 Patient Self-Determination Act   75

6.2 Hospital Policy and Procedures—Patient Self-Determination Act   78

II Medicolegal Forms and Hospital Policies   79

Informed Consent

1.1.1 Hospital Policy and Procedures—Obtaining Informed Consent   81

1.1.2 Informed Consent for Procedures and Operations   85

1.1.3 Consent to the Administration of Anesthesia   86

Refusal of Life-Sustaining Treatment

1.1.4 Jehovah's Witness Refusal of Blood Transfusion and Release   88

1.1.4.1 Optional Clause Where Patient with Minor Children Refuses
Blood   89

1.1.4.2 Second Optional Clause Where Patient with Minor Children
Refuses Blood   89

1.1.5 Refusal of Blood Transfusion (By Patient Who Is Not Jehovah's
Witness)   90

1.2.1 Refusal of Medical Treatment and Release by Patient with
Decision-Making Capacity   91

Refusal of Treatment by Patients With and Without Decision-Making Capacity

1.3.1 Hospital Policy and Procedures—Refusal of Treatment by Patients
with Decision-Making Capacity and by Patients Without
Decision-Making Capacity   93

1.3.1.1 Optional Clause to Expedite Guardianship Proceedings 97

1.3.1.2 Optional Pregnancy Clause   97

1.3.2 Notification to Health Care Surrogate   98

1.3.3 Notification to Proxy   98

1.3.4 Surrogate's, Guardian's, or Proxy's Refusal of Medical Treatment
and Release   99

Right of Refusal and Hospital Policy

1.9.1 Release by Patient Leaving Hospital Against Medical Advice 101

Living Wills

2.3.1 Living Wills: Questions and Answers   102

2.3.2 Living Will (Evaluation of Condition by One Physician) 104

2.3.3 Living Will (Evaluation of Condition by Two Physicians) 105

2.3.4 Direction Concerning the Withholding or Withdrawing of
Artificial Feeding   106

2.3.5 Additional Instructions   106

2.3.6 Optional Pregnancy Clause   106

2.3.7 Direction Concerning Termination of Life Support if Pregnant 107

2.3.8 Revocation   107

Surrogate Decision Making

3.2.1 Advance Directives: Questions and Answers   108

3.2.2 Living Will Designation of Surrogate   110

3.2.3 Advisory for Patients about Health Care Surrogate Designations 110

3.2.4 Health Care Surrogate Designation   111

3.2.4.1 Alternate Health Care Surrogate Designation   112

3.2.4.2 Second Alternate Health Care Surrogate Designation   113

3.2.5 Durable Power of Attorney for Health Care   114

3.2.5.1 Alternate General and Health Care Durable Power of Attorney 115

3.2.5.2 Optional Clause to Determine Principal's Incapacity   116

3.2.5.3 Second Optional Clause to Determine Principal's Incapacity 116

3.2.6 Advance Directive Card for Health Providers   117

3.3.1 Hospital Policy and Procedures—Patients with Advance Directives 118

3.3.2 Affidavit of Close Personal Friend   125

Standards for Surrogate Decision Making

3.4.1 Certification of Adult Terminal Condition and Decision-Making
Capacity   126

Withholding or Withdrawing Life-Sustaining Treatment

4.1.1 Designee's Agreement to Withhold or Withdraw Life Support
After Consultation   128

4.1.1.1 Alternate Request by Surrogate, Guardian, or Proxy to Withhold
or Withdraw Life-Sustaining Procedures   129

4.2.1 Hospital Policy and Procedures—Withholding and Withdrawing
Life-Sustaining Procedures from Adult Terminally Ill Patients   130

4.2.2 Hospital Policy and Procedures—Withholding and Withdrawing
Life-Sustaining Procedures from Pediatric Terminally Ill Patients 138

4.2.3 Certification of Pediatric Terminal Condition   141

4.2.3.1 Alternate Clause Regarding Documentation of Oral Consent by
Proxy for Withholding or Withdrawing Life-Sustaining Treatment from
Pediatric Patient   142

4.2.3.2 Optional Clause Regarding a Minor's Participation in Decision
Making   143

4.2.3.3 Optional Clause to Accept a Minor's Decision to Withhold or
Withdraw Life-Sustaining Treatment   143

4.2.4 Request by Proxy to Withhold or Withdraw Life-Sustaining
Procedures from Pediatric Patient   144

Do-Not-Resuscitate Orders

5.1.1 Cardiopulmonary Resuscitation and Do-Not-Resuscitate Orders:
Questions and Answers   145

5.1.2 Refusal of Cardiopulmonary Resuscitation and Release   147

5.1.3 Consent to No Cardiopulmonary Resuscitation 148

5.1.4 Do-Not-Resuscitate Order 149

5.2.1 Hospital Policy and Procedures—Do-Not-Resuscitate Order 150

5.2.1.1 Optional Clause Permitting Documentation of Oral Refusal of CPR by Surrogate or Proxy 154

5.2.1.2 Do-Not-Resuscitate Progress Notes 155

5.2.1.3 Optional Clause to Expedite Guardianship Proceedings 155

5.2.2 Alternate Hospital Policy and Procedures—Do-Not-Resuscitate Order 156

5.3.1 Prehospital Do-Not-Resuscitate Order 158

Patient Self-Determination Act

6.1.1 Your Rights to Make Health Care Decisions and Advance Directives 162

6.1.2 Advance Directives Brochure 163

6.1.3 Information for Physician's Patients 165

6.1.4 Advance Directive Follow-Up Checklist 166

6.2.1 Hospital Policy and Procedures—Implementation of Patients' Rights Regarding Medical Treatment and Advance Directives 167

Legal Citations 171

References 175

Table of Cases 179

Index 181

Foreword

Since cardiopulmonary resuscitation, a potentially life-saving procedure, was described in 1960 by Dr. Kouwehoven and others, a new era in medicine was launched. In its wake came the artificial prolongation of life in patients in vegetative states, organ transplants, genetic manipulation allowing scientifically assisted conception, and surrogate gestation. These advances in the practice of medicine and the resulting challenges to the mores of society, as well as the ethical dilemmas, were fueled by the media and created a medical-legal vacuum which was quickly filled by attorneys, judges, and the clergy. At present, thirty-three years after the first successful reversal of death, numerous laws, medical-legal forms, hospital policies, consent forms, and so on have been generated. These have proliferated nationwide and expanded in various directions.

Arthur Berger is an attorney, author of a number of books, and a major contributor to the literature on thanatology, religion, and parapsychology. He has written *When Life Ends* to familiarize the medical profession in a field previously neglected by physicians. Today the medical profession, in order to practice modern patient care, requires knowledge of the laws, hospital policies, and available medical-legal forms that govern situations related to near death or end of life. Currently there is nothing in the literature that provides a comprehensive review of the laws and procedures as well as the forms used in this field. This book, by a noted and recognized expert in the field, fills this void and includes noted cases illustrating the many complicated aspects involved in the managed care of the terminally ill. This information is not included in the medical school curriculum or in any of the postgraduate medical programs.

Modern medical care mandates the use of Arthur Berger's *When Life Ends* as required reading in the clinical years of medical school. Recent studies conclude that there is a need for improved communication among physicians, patients, and surrogates, so that decisions for the terminally ill will reflect patients' wishes and best interests. It should be in the library of every hospital and medical school as a ready reference for those in the medical, legal, and clerical fields, as well as the lay public.

Louis Lemberg, M.D.
Professor of Clinical Cardiology
University of Miami School of Medicine

Preface

A fifty-three-year-old female suffering from quadriplegia is alert but helpless and unable to eat or retain solids. A nasogastric tube inserted into her supplies her with nutrition and hydration. With artificial feeding and continued care, she will live for another fifteen or twenty years but she now asks the attending physician to remove the tube. Should the physician accede to the patient's request to terminate life support?

A twenty-seven-year-old plumber with a wife and two minor children is bleeding from a tumor of the colon. His death is certain unless blood is administered to him, but he refuses it because he is a Jehovah's Witness. Should the hospital apply for a court order to compel the Jehovah's Witness to receive a blood transfusion?

A middle-aged bachelor with no family has developed renal failure and cardiomyopathy and is in need of dialysis. But his decision-making capacity is in serious question. A male friend to whom the patient has left the bulk of his large estate comes forward with a living will signed by the patient in which the friend has been named proxy. The friend directs the attending physician to withhold dialysis. Must dialysis be withheld because the proxy has requested it, or should the proxy's motive and possible conflict of interest be questioned?

An attending doctor sees no reasonable hope of survival for a seventy-year-old male patient with asystole electromechanical dissociation. The physician writes a do-not-resuscitate order because in her judgment cardiopulmonary resuscitation would be futile and inhumane therapy. Is she permitted to write and enter in the patient's medical record a do-not-resuscitate order without talking with or getting the consent of the patient?

These dramas and the issues they raise are some of the many kinds of dramas and issues that are played out inevitably and constantly on the stage of medical decision making when a patient's life is at or near its end. The dramas such as those described raise specific questions pertinent to their particular circumstances. But certain key questions cut across all dramas and, like playful porpoises, keep surfacing again and again whenever and wherever hospital ethics committees (such as the one on which I serve), physicians, or hospital legal counsel are called on to make end-of-life decisions: "What does the law say?" "Have we designed a form to cover this?" "Has a policy been developed for this situation?" "What is the procedure to be followed here?"

This book was written in response to a need to address these common and legitimate concerns. It is the first comprehensive compilation of the law, medicolegal forms, and hospital policies and procedures applicable to end-of-life matters.

The purpose of the book will be served if it is used as an aid by hospitals, nursing homes, medical records managers, physicians, registered nurses, students of medicine and nursing, and others whose professional duties require them to care for and work with the dying patient. With its collection of medicolegal forms, and hospital policies on such matters as informed consent, refusal of medical treatment, advance directives, surrogate decision making, withholding and withdrawing of life-sustaining treatment, do-not-resuscitate orders, and the Patient Self-Determination Act, the book may also be valuable as a resource for health law attorneys and hospital ethics committees or consultants concerned with complex issues in patient care.

According to the U.S. National Center for Health Statistics, 2.2 million Americans die every year. Of these, 80 percent die in hospitals or nursing homes. Although this book is intended primarily for care givers, the essential information it contains relating to legal and ethical issues in end-of-life care should also attract the interest and attention of the eight out of ten of us who will become care receivers in the institutions in which we die.

Introduction

Until recently, physicians could do no more for their patients than treat symptoms, inject morphine, and give oxygen. They would tell their patients: "There is nothing more that I or medicine can do for you." Only nature and time were the real physicians who might effect cures. But today advances in medical technology have expanded the therapeutic arsenal and given physicians new power. Remarkable and dramatic as these advances are, they make some of us wonder: "[F]or the first time in history, physicians have the ability, know-how and sophisticated technology to sustain the physical life of patients beyond any reasonable quality of life they might want to endure. What does that mean?" (Scully and Scully, 1987:16).

There is no single meaning. There are several that apply to *end-of-life matters*, a term used to refer to various aspects of the six subjects listed in the Table of Contents: refusal of life-sustaining treatment, living wills, surrogate decision making, withholding and withdrawing life-sustaining treatment, the do-not-resuscitate order, and the Patient Self-Determination Act.

We make a start toward discovering these meanings by observing that, in the wake of medical advances, numerous legal problems were raised with which lawmakers were forced to deal for the first time. Most of us picture, and even reliable dictionaries are prone to define, a *lawmaker* as a legislator. But those who make laws are not necessarily our elected representatives in Congress or in the state legislatures, whose statutes make up the written law. The "lawmaker" is also the judge who makes the equally powerful common or unwritten law based on custom, the decisions of other judges, or learned treatises, or in response to factual situations presenting novel issues not covered by the existing written law.

In 1975 such a situation took shape and wriggled through a courtroom door because of a mistake. A twenty-one-year-old woman took drugs and alcohol, went into a coma, and was rushed to a New Jersey hospital. Although functioning, her brain was damaged, she was in a persistent vegetative condition, and a life-support apparatus was administered to her. Convinced that their daughter would never emerge into a cognitive state, her parents asked the physicians and hospital to take their daughter off the mechanical respirator that was artificially maintaining her life. When they refused, the parents committed their error. They did not make use of the simple expedients of changing physicians or transferring their daughter to another hospital. Instead the parents went to court by filing a complaint in the chancery division of superior court, asking that the patient be declared incompetent and that her father be appointed legal guardian with power to discontinue all extraordinary means of sustaining his daughter's life.

The daughter's name was Karen Ann Quinlan. The superior court refused the parents' petition because it said that the matter should be left to the medical profession. The father then appealed to the New Jersey Supreme Court, which reversed the lower court in 1976 and granted the petition. Its ruling in *In re Quinlan*[1] was a landmark decision in several respects. The one to be noted here is that it took the resolution of end-of-life issues out of the hands of physicians and delivered them to the courts to decide. The case challenged the monopoly of the medical profession over end-of-life matters and ended the long-established authority of physicians to make decisions whether to keep alive patients in Karen's condition.

The importance of this case cannot be overstated. One consequence of it was that courts and legislators assumed the principal role as mediator in controversies over end-of-life issues between patients and their families on one side and physicians and hospitals on the other. Jurisprudence—not medicine, philosophy, ethics, or religion—became the real-life decision maker. The first meaning of medical advances is this: Next to medical knowledge and expertise, no information has become more in demand when medical decisions are made near or at life's end than judicial decisions and statutes. More than any other force in society, the law enunciated by the courts and legislatures in this area plays the supreme role in resolving disputes between patient and health provider and in addressing needs created by developments in medical technology. It is on their statutes and case law that health professionals and patients depend almost daily for their guidance and with which they need to become familiar.

A second meaning of advances in medicine is that end-of-life issues were created by them, which produced and continue to produce conflicts over what is "right," "wrong," or "legal."

A third meaning is that, as one commentator on health law has said, "American medicine is awash in forms" (Annas, 1991:1210) and that, in the end-of-life field, hospitals, physicians, and attorneys need to become informed and updated about the medicolegal forms necessitated by the new developments in medicine and the changing face of the law.

A final meaning is that health facilities need to develop and implement policies and procedures in keeping with end-of-life medical and legal developments.

These meanings alone justify this book, which deals with them. It is organized to be useful and informative in two ways. First, it assumes that health professionals do not have either the time or the opportunity to plunge into the legal and medical literature, or to consult with legal counsel to understand or update the law relative to an end-of-life situation, or to rummage through filing cabinets filled with forms in order to locate desired documents. Next best to having an attorney look over one's shoulder or poring through paperwork is this book, which is designed as a quick information resource to make frequently raised legal and ethical issues and important forms and procedures readily available to readers at a minimum of effort. Three devices have been used to help readers easily and quickly locate what is desired. The Table of Contents pinpoints exactly where a particular topic with its legal analysis and institutional procedures is discussed. The forms are listed with topical headings and numbered to pinpoint the sections of the text where medicolegal forms and institutional policies are to be found. A detailed index permits readers to find any item sought.

Second, *When Life Ends* contains sections in which will be found legal citations and references to further sources of information and which consist of legal analyses interwoven with legal and ethical issues, forms, and institutional policies and procedures.

LEGAL OVERVIEWS

There is ample reason to believe that health professionals do not understand or are puzzled over the legal principles applicable to the end-of-life situations they must encounter. The do-not-resuscitate order, for example, presents one of the most troublesome situations in medical practice. "That's terrible!" groaned a physician of my acquaintance when she learned that doctors in another hospital had made unilateral decisions to withhold cardiopulmonary resuscitation for some patients and, after they had written do-not-resuscitate orders, stopped all care for the patients. "Those physicians really need to be educated," she added. Studies suggest that she is right because "confusion with respect to these orders is so great" (Mittelberger et al., 1993:228).

Professional ignorance of or confusion about the law applicable close to or at the end of a life can lead not only to inappropriate patient care but also to patient anguish and anger. An incident in 1989 provided one example. Physicians at Rush Presbyterian-St. Luke's Hospital in Illinois misunderstood or were uncertain about whether life-sustaining treatment could be legally withdrawn from a patient who was not "brain dead." Frustrated by their refusal to withdraw life-sustaining treatment from his comatose infant son after he pleaded with them, the father himself unplugged the respirator from the child while he held the staff at gunpoint ("Questions of Law," 1989). In still another instructive case, physicians refused to withdraw life-sustaining treatment from a patient who was "brain dead" and to turn his body over to his parents; the parents promptly sued them for the tort of outrage and recovered.[2]

As one noted authority said, "Doctors don't know the law" (Annas, 1988:621). There is a clear need to educate them about it. To this end, my prior book (Berger, 1993) brought together case and statutory law applicable to dying patients, the right to die, advance directives, brain death, and organ transplantation and assembled them into a "law of dying and death." The fresh contribution of *When Life Ends* to this educational process consists of several new elements. First are its extensive legal overviews. The book, of course, is not intended to provide legal counsel as to the law presently existing in a given state. Since the law is always in a state of flux and amendments to statutes are constant, readers should consult the statutes or attorneys in their states for specific factual situations and issues. The intention, however, is to supply general legal information and to do so in a manner resembling a tour taken by visitors to strange and exotic places. After they have gone to all the popular tourist sites, eventually they find a high vantage point which gives them a panoramic and unforgettable view of everything. The legal overviews offer a sweeping survey of all the legal points of special interest relative to end-of-life matters. Identified will be subjects and pertinent issues which have been sparked by the growth of biomedical knowledge and techniques. Some of these subjects and issues, which continue to divide and be debated by health professionals, lawyers, philosophers, and theologians, include the following.

Refusal of Life-Sustaining Treatment

Is there a right to refuse life-sustaining treatment? If there is, what supports it? What are the interests of the state and is the right outweighed by these interests? Is the right limited to terminally ill patients? Is it limited to treatment that is extraordinary? Is it limited to treatment that has not been started? Does it extend to artificial nutrition and hydration? Does it extend to asking physicians to aid suffering patients to die? Do policies of health care facilities outweigh it? Should health professionals be forced to give treatment which violates their beliefs? Is confirmation by a court needed for decisions to discontinue or not to start life-sustaining treatment?

Advance Directives

What are they? What provisions are shared in common by living will statutes? What are the types, form, and content of advance directives? Why and how should they be made?

Surrogate Decision Making

Are patients lacking decision-making capacity denied the right to accept or reject treatment? What is decision-making capacity? Who may make decisions for patients lacking decision-making capacity? What restrictions are placed on these decisions? By what standards are these decisions made? What is the decision-making process?

Withholding or Withdrawing Life-Sustaining Treatment

For a patient without decision-making capacity, when and by whom may the decision be made to terminate life-sustaining treatment? What are the examinations to be made and procedures to be followed for terminating life support for adult patients? For minor patients?

Do-Not-Resuscitate Orders

What is a do-not-resuscitate order? May it be issued on the ground that CPR is futile? What does "futility" mean? Who is to make the final decision whether CPR is to be withheld: physician or patient? What is a prehospital do-not-resuscitate order?

Patient Self-Determination Act

What is the aim of the act? What are health facilities required to do to meet its requirements?

FORMS

Another fresh element in this book is its forms incorporated by reference into the legal overviews. The term *forms* is intended to cover medical or legal documents that are used regularly in the practice of medicine in connection with end-of-life matters. Such documents may express patients' rights, directions, or wishes, inform patients, contain physicians' documentations, or establish hospital policies or procedures.

The forms used in medicine never saved a patient's life. They are generally condemned as making medicine routinized and bureaucratic and are shunned by many physicians and nurses as a colossal bore and burden that take up too much of their time and interfere with professional responsibilities. Some may even object, "I am a health professional taking care of patients, not a clerk giving out or filling out forms." But we cannot do without forms. They provide important practical tools for handling problems and serving needs in patient care.

Forms have two kinds of legal importance. They can advise patients of their legal rights and help them and their families protect these rights. In addition, forms are admissible as evidence in litigation against a physician or a hospital, say for withdrawing life support or not doing so in defiance of a patient's wishes. In such cases, failure to maintain the proper forms may result in civil or criminal liability. On the other hand, forms that are complete and accurate can contribute to a successful defense by showing that what was done or not done to a patient was reasonable and proper.

As will be seen from the list of forms in the Table of Contents, the sections of the book contain a variety of valuable end-of-life documents pertaining to informed consent, refusal of and withholding or withdrawing of life-sustaining treatment, advance directives, surrogate decision making, do-not-resuscitate orders, and the Patient Self-Determination Act. Over seventy such forms are provided. Many bear the seal of authority. Some were adapted from state statutes, some were taken from the records of court cases in which the provisions of an instrument were the focus of judicial approval, and some were the products of careful deliberations by the ethics committee of a large medical center.

All the forms are basic ones that should be useful as samples in most situations. Since both medicine and the law are always changing and unusual conditions may arise, the forms may serve as beginning points for the preparation of other documents that may be required. Since no forms can be drafted to meet every need or problem, some alternate forms are provided, as are alternate and optional clauses that may be used to adapt a basic form. The forms are suggestive only and may not be valid in the reader's state. Before using the forms in a particular state, one must take care, therefore, to conform them to the law of that state, since the validity of an instrument and the rights it creates may be determined by the law of the state in which it is executed and in which the rights arise.

A numbering system has been used for the subjects and sections of the book. For example, "Surrogate Decision Making" is number 3 and its sections are numbered 3.1, 3.2, 3.3, and 3.4. Similarly, a numbering system is used for the forms. Each is given the number of the subject to which the form is pertinent, followed by a decimal point, followed by the number of the section which discusses it, followed by a decimal point, then the number of the form. Thus, a form for a durable power of attorney for health care is identified as 3.2.5; 3 relates to surrogate decision making, 2 refers to the section in which the form appears, and 5 is the form number. If alternate forms or optional clauses are suggested, they will be identified in the same manner except that there will be a third decimal point followed by the number of the alternate form or optional clause. Thus, in section 3.2, an alternate form for a durable power of attorney for health care would be 3.2.5.1, and an optional clause for the basic form would be 3.2.5.2.

HOSPITAL POLICIES AND PROCEDURES

We need to recognize as well that patient care and the decisions of health care providers about treatment are governed not only by the law. They are also guided by the written policies and procedures developed by hospitals and long-term care facilities. A legal commentator once made the comparison between legislators and parties to a contract. The legislators pass laws to create the rights and duties of the people they represent, and the contracting parties create their own rights and duties by virtue of their contract (Cohen, 1933). Health care institutions similarly create the rights and duties of all those working or residing in them with the policies they create. Hospital policies and protocols are, therefore, important, and different ones must be formulated to address different medical situations. Accordingly, another element of *When Life Ends* is the hospital policies and procedures which accompany the legal overviews and which address procedures for obtaining informed consent; refusal of treatment by patients with and without decision-making capacity; withholding or withdrawing life-sustaining treatment from adult terminally ill patients and from pediatric terminally ill patients; do-not-resuscitate orders; and implementation of patients' rights regarding medical treatment and advance directives in accordance with the Patient Self-Determination Act.

Many of the policies and procedures incorporated into the legal overviews were established and implemented by a 750-bed public hospital which annually admits 24,000 patients. It should not be inferred from this, however, that only large hospitals require policies and procedures to meet legal and ethical end-of-life issues. The life-and-death decisions made by or on behalf of patients in a hospital with 20 beds are no less important than those made by or on behalf of a patient in a 750-bed hospital. Nor should it be inferred that the policies supplied are permanent and inflexible. They may be suggestive for physicians and hospitals who may wish to adopt different policies. It is hoped that these materials will supply guidelines as well as practical tools for the staffs of small and large hospitals, and long-term care facilities and individual practitioners, for better patient care, and for medical practice that conforms to the law applicable when life ends.

LEGAL CITATIONS

1. In re Quinlan, 70 N.J. 10, 355 A.2d 647 (N.J. Supreme Court) *cert. den. sub. nom.* In re Garger v. New Jersey, 429 U.S. 922 (1976).

2. Strachan v. John F. Kennedy Memorial Hospital, 209 N.J. Superior Court 300, 507 A.2d 718, *aff'd* in part, 109 N.J. 523, 538 A.2d 346 (N.J. Supreme Ct. 1988).

REFERENCES

Annas, George J. 1991. "The Health Care Proxy and the Living Will." *New England Journal of Medicine* 324:1210–1213.
——— . 1988. "The Paradoxes of Organ Transplantation." *American Journal of Public Health* 78:621–622.
Berger, A. S. 1993. *Dying and Death in Law and Medicine: A Forensic Primer for Health and Legal Professionals.* Westport, CT: Praeger.
Cohen, Morris R. 1933. "The Basis of Contract." *Harvard Law Review* 46:553–592, at 586.
Mittelberger, J. A., Lo, B., Martin, D., and Uhlmann, R. F. 1993. "Impact of a Procedure-Specific Do Not Resuscitate Order Form on Documentation of Do Not Resuscitate Orders." *Archives of Internal Medicine* 153:228–232.
"Questions of Law Live on after Father Helps Son Die." 1989. *New York Times,* 7 May, p. 26, col. 1.
Scully, T., and Scully, C. 1987. *Playing God: The New World of Medical Choices.* New York: Simon and Schuster.

I

LEGAL OVERVIEWS

1

Refusal of
Life-Sustaining Treatment

1.1 RIGHT TO REFUSE LIFE-SUSTAINING TREATMENT

Forty-nine-year-old Paul Brophy was a patient in New England Mt. Sinai Hospital in Massachusetts. He had been a firefighter and medical technician before his operation for an aneurysm that produced a brain hemorrhage. Following surgery, he entered into a persistent vegetative state. Although he was not terminally ill, he was unable to swallow, and a gastrostomy tube was inserted into his stomach to provide him with food and water. Brophy had once told his wife, Patricia, when they were talking about the case of Karen Ann Quinlan, "I don't ever want to be on a life-support system. No way do I want to live like that; that is not living." Now, as she recalled what he said, Patricia Brophy agonized over whether his life support should be terminated.

This same scenario parades past us in an endless army of clones as it continues to take place in every hospital every day. The days of patients in Brophy's tragic situation, like his days, are over but their suns are prevented from setting by mechanical means which sustain their vital functions and keep them alive as mindless beings incapable of social interaction. These recurring scenes force us into confrontation with religious values and economic as well as ethical issues (Berger, 1993:52–69), as patients rebel against medical miracles which would prolong their merely biological, vegetative existences.

Physicians may accept patient autonomy intellectually but nevertheless concerns welling up deep within them force doctors to see the decisions of patients or their families to withhold or withdraw life support as "wrong." These concerns include uncertainty about the legal consequences that may result from a too easy acquiescence in these decisions, a strong belief in the role a physician should play, and, perhaps most strongly, the fear that honoring the patient's or family's wish will result in killing the patient as opposed to letting the patient die (Fried et al., 1993). Thus, when, after much reflection, prayer, and discussion with her family and the clergy, Patricia Brophy decided that her husband's life was over and asked for the removal of the tube from her husband, the attending physician, the hospital medical staff, and the board of directors of the hospital all concurred in refusing to carry out her request because of their moral conviction that they would be killing Brophy.

The artificial maintenance of physical life also signifies the creation of substantive and procedural legal issues whose sensitivity and difficulty are highlighted by the reported appellate decisions. Faced with the refusal of the hospital to accede to her wishes, Patricia Brophy carried her case into the courts of Massachusetts to ask that her husband be allowed to die. It reached the high court of the state, whose final ruling was by a split decision with three of the seven judges dissenting from the majority view.[1] The Massachusetts case is not unique in demonstrating a lack of judicial unanimity in cases involving decisions whether or not to terminate life-sustaining treatment. Famous illustrations are the recent decisions by split courts in the case of Nancy Cruzan—5–4 in the U.S. Supreme Court and 4–3 in the Missouri Supreme Court.[2] These are joined by many other major court decisions[3] which also have either reversed lower or appellate courts, as happened in *Brophy,* or which were not unanimous in the high courts, again as in *Brophy.* This case acts as a mirror for every case in that perplexing and demanding region of law in which a court is called on to decide whether a patient will be permitted to die.

Brophy acts as well as a springboard for posing the following legal questions posed in this section and in sections 1.2, 1.4, and 1.5 through 1.11. *Does a competent adult who objects to life-sustaining treatment have the right to refuse it even if that refusal means death?* A long line of court decisions clearly recognize the right of a patient to accept or reject medical treatment. The right is grounded in several alternate basic societal, common-law, and constitutional concepts: self-determination, informed consent, privacy, liberty interest, and religious beliefs.

Self-Determination and Informed Consent

A fundamental principle governs American society and should govern the dealings between society and the individual. John Stuart Mill expressed the principle as self-protection:

[T]he only purpose for which power can be rightfully exercised over any member of the civilized community, against his will, is to prevent harm to others. His own good, either physical or moral, is not a sufficient warrant. . . . The only part of the conduct of anyone, for which he is amenable to society, is that which concerns others. In the part which merely concerns himself, his independence is, of right, absolute. Over himself, over his own body and mind, the individual is sovereign. (Mill, 1961:484)

That judicial decisions have long recognized the concept of individual self-determination and its relation to medical treatment is shown in the following quotations:

Anglo-American law starts with the premise of thoroughgoing self-determination. It follows that each man is considered to be the master of his own body, and he may, if he be of sound mind, expressly prohibit the performance of life-saving surgery or other medical treatment.[4]

[N]o right is held more sacred, or is more carefully guarded by the common law, than the right of every individual to the possession and control of his own person, free of all restraint and interference of others, unless by clear and unquestionable authority and the law.[5]

Under a free government at least, the free citizen's first and greatest right which underlies all others—the right to the inviolability of his person, in other words his right to himself—is the subject of universal acquiescence, and this right necessarily forbids a physician . . . to violate without permission the bodily integrity of his patient by a major or capital operation.[6]

Every human being of adult years and sound mind has a right to determine what shall be done with his own body; and a surgeon who performs an operation without his patient's consent commits an assault for which he is liable in damages.[7]

The doctrine of informed consent emerged in the courts from the tort law of assault—the apprehension of contact with someone's person without consent—and battery—the actual and intentional contact—and to protect the autonomy of the individual and one's interest in the inviolability of one's body. Founded on these common-law concepts and the rights of individuals to consent voluntarily and without coercion before any contact is made with their bodies, the doctrine forces a physician to make disclosures to a patient concerning a proposed treatment or procedure in order that any consent to the touching of the patient's body will be based on full medical information. Patients are to be informed about their diagnoses, the nature of the proposed treatment or procedure, its benefits and risks, alternative therapies and their benefits and risks, what may happen during the recuperation process after the procedure or treatment, and what may happen if the proposed course of action is not followed. Failure to obtain consent for a procedure may give rise to liability for a battery. Performing a procedure after obtaining consent based on failure of a physician to provide complete information about the procedure so that the consent is not an "informed consent" may create liability for professional negligence or malpractice.

Since the doctrine of informed consent is central to the physician-patient relationship, it would seem to require the formulation of a hospital policy. **Form 1.1.1** suggests a policy which recognizes that all health care is predicated on it.

The policy spells out the obligation of medical professionals, before initiating procedures, to obtain informed consent from a patient. If the patient's decision-making capacity is lacking or impaired and the patient has made no advance directive, medical professionals must get consent from the patient's health care surrogate (someone designated by the patient to make health care decisions in the event of the patient's incapacity to make them) or from the patient's legitimate proxy (if the surrogate is not available or cannot or will not perform the duties of a surrogate). No prior consent need be obtained, however, in an emergency when a patient's medical condition requires the taking of immediate measures to sustain the life of a patient or to save the patient's health from being permanently damaged and when, because of the emergency, the patient's consent or that of people authorized to act for the patient cannot be obtained. The policy also specifies the following: (1) by whom and how a consent must be signed. Unless a consent is in the language of the patient, it should provide that a consent should contain the interpreter's name and that the interpreter should sign it as well as a registered nurse acting as a witness; (2) the contents of the consent; (3) that the patient, surrogate, or proxy received an explanation from the relevant health professional concerning the proposed treatment, the likely risks and benefits, and possible alternative medical treatments, including the option of refusal and its risks and consequences; and (4) that the patient, surrogate, or proxy was able to ask questions of those charged with the care of the patient.

For an adult patient for whom a surrogate has not been designated or is not able or willing to act, the proxy generally is selected according to the following order of priority: a legal guardian appointed previously with authority to consent to medical treatment; the spouse; an adult child or a majority of the adult children; the parents; an adult sibling or a majority of the adult siblings; an adult relative familiar with the patient's beliefs; or a close personal friend, an adult who has maintained regular contact with the patient and is willing to be involved with the patient's medical care. If the hospital cannot find a surrogate or proxy, it may be required to petition a court to determine its authority and duty. The policy calls for notification to be given to legal counsel in these circumstances.

An adult is one who has reached the age of majority, in some states the age of eighteen, and in others the age of twenty-one. Under that age, an individual does not have the capacity to consent to treatment unless, by the statute of a particular state, the person is emancipated—someone not under parental custody and living independently and taking care of his or her own affairs, married, or in the armed services. For an underage and unemancipated patient, the consent to medical treatment of a legitimate proxy would be needed—first the legal guardian, then the one who has authority to consent to medical treatment, then the natural or adoptive parents, and finally, the nearest adult relative.

Absent judicial approval or express authority from a patient, health care surrogates and proxies, however, are not empowered to consent to certain procedures, including abortion, sterilization, experimental treatments that do not have the approval of an institutional review board concerned with protecting the rights of human subjects in compliance with the Code of Federal Regulations, and the withholding or withdrawing of life-sustaining procedures from a pregnant patient prior to viability of the fetus.

Two forms of consent are generally obtained from patients prior to initiating any procedures. The first is a general consent signed when entering a hospital. It relates to routine hospital and nursing services and noninvasive diagnostic procedures and is to be placed in the patient's chart. In addition to the admission consent form, hospitals and physicians use a special consent form for special or invasive diagnostic and surgical procedures. Form 1.1.2 proposes a form of special consent to be obtained from and signed by a patient or, if the patient lacks decision-making capacity, by a health care surrogate or proxy to authorize a stipulated operation or procedure. The consent form, to be signed also by a witness and interpreter, if needed, contains an acknowledgment that an explanation has been given concerning the method of procedure, the risks and benefits of the contemplated treatment, the alternatives and their risks, and the risks connected with refusal. The consent also covers the admission of observers and the taking of pictures during the course of the procedure or operation.

Form 1.1.3 supplies a consent to the administration of anesthesia. In it, a patient acknowledges that it is the anesthesiologist, and not the surgeon, who administers the anesthesia and who decides which forms of anesthesia can be used. The patient consents to one method but authorizes use of a different one if unforeseen conditions arise. The patient also acknowledges an understanding of the possible complications that may arise and assumes the risk of anesthesia. The form is to be signed by the patient, surrogate, or proxy, the interpreter (if one is necessary), and a witness and countersigned by the anesthesiologist.

Since every competent adult individual has the right to self-determination and bodily integrity and the right to consent to treatment, the corollary of the informed consent doctrine is that an individual has the right not to consent, that is, to refuse medical treatment in spite of the fact that refusal will cause great risk to health or even hasten death. *Matter of Claire Conroy* and other court decisions[8] have used the doctrine as the ground for the right to refuse treatment variously described as "life-saving," "life-prolonging," or "life-sustaining." But these are confusing terms. Does it matter whether a life has been saved, prolonged, or sustained? *Life-sustaining treatment*, the term used in this book, does not include medications or medical procedures needed to alleviate pain or provide comfort care. It is generally understood to embrace any medical procedure, treatment, or intervention which utilizes mechanical or other artificial means to sustain or replace a spontaneous vital function and, in the case of a terminally ill patient, serves only to prolong the dying process. The patient's right to refuse it is protected even if the refusal conflicts with what medical judgment deems necessary to save the life of the patient. The patient is the final arbiter, and the law does not allow physicians to substitute their judgments for that of the patient.

Privacy

A right to privacy or what is called the right to be let alone was recognized by the U.S. Supreme Court in *Griswold v. Connecticut*.[9] Although the U.S. Constitution did not expressly confer this right, the nation's high court in *Roe v. Wade*[10] interpreted the Fourteenth Amendment as creating it and observed that courts or individual justices had also pointed to the First, Fourth, Fifth, and Ninth Amendments as well as the Bill of Rights as its sources. This right has been construed as giving autonomy in many areas. It is really a bundle of rights, such as the right not to be spied on in our bedrooms, not to have our phone conversations listened to (at least not without a court order), and not to have our photographs used in advertising. The right of privacy also gives us the right to make intimate choices. Thus, the U.S. Supreme Court extended it to procreation decisions, such as whether to use contraception (as in *Griswold*) or to have an abortion (as in *Roe v. Wade*). But it had never recognized medical decisions or the right to refuse treatment as embodied in the right to privacy, nor had any state court. Therefore, in the case of *In re Quinlan*,[11] the New Jersey Supreme Court's holding—that the right to privacy is also "broad enough to encompass a patient's decision to decline medical treatment" and thereby to end a life that is no longer worth living and that has no prospect of returning to a cognitive state—was a landmark. It was the first authority for the principle that although the U.S. Constitution does not specifically give the right to die, it does support treatment refusal. Following *Quinlan*, the privacy right was thereafter used by many state courts as a basis for treatment refusal.[12] The *Brophy* court, for example, which decided that Patricia Brophy's wishes to have her husband's feeding tube removed must be respected, held that "a significant aspect of this right of privacy is the right to be free of nonconsensual invasion of one's bodily integrity."[13]

Liberty Interest

The case of *Cruzan v. Director, Missouri Department of Health*[14] was of great importance because the U.S. Supreme Court had never directly addressed the constitutional right of a person to refuse life-sustaining treatment. It focused national attention on the issue of termination of life-sustaining treatment. With Chief Justice William Rehnquist writing the opinion and describing the case as entailing the right to die, the majority of the court held that under the federal Constitution a competent adult has a right to refuse life-sustaining treatment. The majority declined to extend the constitutional privacy right past the begetting of children and to extend it to include treatment refusal, as some state courts had done. It also declined to base its holding on the autonomy of the individual, which the common law so zealously guarded. Instead, the majority viewed an unwanted bodily invasion as representing an interference with the liberty of the individual. Some commentators interpret the Supreme Court's decision as based on "the right of liberty" (Weir and Gostin, 1990:1848), but the Court did not use this language. It preferred to analyze treatment refusal as a "liberty interest" under the Fourteenth Amendment of the federal Constitution, which prohibits a state from arbitrarily depriving an individual of life, liberty, or property without due process of law. In so doing the high court carved out of the Constitution a new interest and bent the document to fit the times and developments in medical technology. The due process clause became another basis for the right to die.

Religious Beliefs

Up until 1976 when the *Quinlan* case was decided, there were few cases concerned with the termination of life-sustaining treatment. The pre-1976 cases in which patients refused life-sustaining treatment did not involve those matters of which we hear so much today—autonomy, informed consent, privacy, liberty—because the grounds of their refusals were religious beliefs based on scripture. These were the cases of Jehovah's Witnesses who, because they believe that it is forbidden by the Bible, will not accept homologous or autologous whole blood, packed red blood cells, packed white blood cells, or platelets. Since the number of Witnesses and their associates in the United States is increasing, physicians and hospitals can expect to continue to encounter the ethical and legal issues they present.

There is no doubt that their refusal of blood creates a problem for physicians committed to applying their medical expertise and technology to the prolongation of life. Jehovah's Witnesses seem to understand this and ask that, instead of considering them a problem, physicians accept the Witnesses as a medical challenge (Dixon and Smalley, 1981).

The legal issues presented by Jehovah's Witnesses include these two questions: When a Witness on religious grounds refuses a blood transfusion even if it means death, is a court authorized to step in and decide for the Witness? Do people have a right to die for their religious beliefs?

In these cases, the important clause of the U.S. Constitution is the First Amendment, which provides that "Congress shall make no law . . . prohibiting the free exercise" of religion. This provision is made applicable to the states by the Fourteenth Amendment. Therefore, in the well-known case of *In re Brooks*,[15] where a Jehovah's Witness without minor children refused a blood transfusion, the court decided it could not interfere notwithstanding its belief that the woman's decision was "foolish and unwise." The First Amendment conferred the right to exercise religious beliefs and since there was here no threat to the morals, welfare, or health of society and no minor children, there was no ground for judicial intervention. In these cases of childless adults, the free exercise clause of the U.S. Constitution is unqualified, admits of no exceptions, and is the basis for the right to die.

Normally, a patient's religious beliefs are of no consequence to health care providers and have no effect on patient care. If these beliefs impel patients with decision-making capacity to refuse treatment, hospital policies that recognize patient autonomy, such as the one given below in **Form 1.3.1**, will govern such situations. In every case, as where a Jehovah's Witness refuses a blood transfusion, a written refusal and release should be completed to protect the hospital and health care provider from charges of neglect to provide the treatment. The refusal should also be noted in the patient's chart. Jehovah's Witnesses seem ready enough to accept full responsibility for their refusals of blood and to relieve physicians and health care facilities from liability, and they will generally sign blood refusal forms when admitted to the hospital. Form 1.1.4 suggests a refusal of blood transfusion by a Witness together with a release to medical personnel and hospital for injury or death which may result therefrom. The form is to be signed by the patient, two witnesses, and by the attending physician.

Cases in which Jehovah's Witnesses with minor children for whom there is no provision for their welfare refuse blood create considerable uncertainty for a hospital about its duties and frequently force it to petition a court for an order determining its responsibilities. One of two alternative policies might alleviate the situation. If a hospital wants to override a patient's wishes in order to assert the state's interest in protecting a minor child, Form 1.1.4.1 provides an optional clause to be inserted in Form 1.1.4. But if a hospital does not wish to stand in the way of the wishes of its patient in favor of nonpatients and prefers to have the state bear the burden of protecting its own interests, Form 1.1.4.2 provides a second optional clause that might be placed in Form 1.1.4.

Form 1.1.4 is designed specifically for Jehovah's Witnesses. Form 1.1.5 is provided for those with convictions, religious or otherwise, against the acceptance of blood.

Cases of minor children who do not receive medical treatment because of their parents' religious beliefs test the strength of the free-exercise clause and raise the constitutional issue of whether the right to exercise religious beliefs is absolute. It is generally held by courts[16] that, under the guise of religious beliefs, parents cannot be relieved of the care of their children. The holdings show that there are limitations on the right to exercise religious beliefs. It is not absolute when state interests are endangered. Where children are involved, the interest of society is to protect them, and the state, as *parens patriae* (i.e., "father of the country") and legal guardian and protector of children and incompetents, will infringe the religious rights of parents.

1.2 RIGHT OF REFUSAL AND STATE INTERESTS

Can the interests of the state be used to override a patient's right to refuse life-sustaining treatment? With the informed consent doctrine standing guard over patients, their freedom from unwanted treatment seems to be guaranteed. But such is not the case because zealous state attorneys general and not a few physicians and hospitals have succeeded in convincing courts to use one of the four overriding interests of the state to issue orders coercing treatment:

prevention of suicide, protection of innocent third parties, the ethics of the medical profession, and the preservation of life.

Prevention of Suicide

Actual suicide at one time was a felony in England but today there as well as in the United States suicide has been decriminalized. Attempting to take one's own life, however, remains criminal in some jurisdictions. In these as well as in those states where it is not a crime, the state has intervened in some cases to order life-sustaining treatment in the face of objection by a competent adult. The most widely cited case in which this was done is *John F. Kennedy Memorial Hospital v. Heston*,[17] where a twenty-two-year-old unmarried woman refused a blood transfusion because she was a Jehovah's Witness. She was forced to have one anyway on the theory that there is no difference between passively submitting to death and actively seeking it. The state regards both as attempts at self-destruction and may prevent them. Since this case, however, the trend of cases has been away from this reasoning and toward subordinating the state's interest in the prevention of suicide to the rights of patients to forgo or have withdrawn life-sustaining treatment. *Brophy* offers one reason. Discontinuance of Brophy's gastrostomy tube was not the death-producing agent set in motion by the patient with the intent of causing death. When death occurs as a result of discontinuing life support, it occurs because of natural causes. Other cases are in accord with this approach.[18] A further reason is that since competent adults have the common-law and constitutional right to accept or decline medical treatment, they cannot be subjected to criminal liability for attempting suicide when they try to exercise the right.[19]

Protection of Third Parties

Courts have intervened on the ground of the state's interest in the protection of innocent parties, specifically, minor children. There are two general types of cases in this category. One situation is where a parent asserts a religious belief as a reason for refusing medical treatment for a child. In such a case, the state as *parens patriae* will step in to see that the child receives needed treatment in spite of the parents' religious beliefs.[20] In a second situation, a parent with a child under eighteen years of age may try to refuse life-sustaining treatment. In such a case, some courts have intervened to order treatment for the unwilling parent. On the basis of the doctrine of *parens patriae*, the state will sometimes seek to prevent minor children from being abandoned. Thus, one judge would not permit the mother of a minor child to refuse blood and to die because death was the ultimate abandonment.[21] In other cases, however, it seems clear that the *parens patriae* doctrine does not require that a child be reared by two parents instead of one. If one parent of a minor child refuses on religious grounds to have a blood transfusion that would save the life of the parent but the child would be cared for and reared by another parent with the aid of immediate members of the family, there is not enough evidence of abandonment to support the state's claim that minor children must be protected. The state will therefore not be permitted to override the constitutional right of free religious exercise by the first parent.[22]

Ethics of the Medical Profession

Courts often acknowledge that one of the interests of the state is the maintenance of the ethical standards of the medical profession and the safeguarding of its integrity. On the basis of this interest, hospitals and physicians argue that they have the right to provide the patient all necessary and appropriate medical treatment. However, like the state's interest in preventing suicide, this one is not endangered by allowing a patient to refuse life-sustaining treatment. As one court said, "If the patient's right to informed consent is to have any meaning at all, it must be accorded respect even when it conflicts with the advice of the doctor or the values of the medical profession as a whole."[23] However, this does not necessarily signify that the integrity of the medical profession will be ignored or that it will be coerced into performing affirmative acts that violate its values. For a further discussion of this point, see Section 1.10.

Preservation of Life

This is the most powerful of the state's interests. But recent cases have not allowed it to override the right of competent patients to refuse treatment. For example, in *Quinlan* a respirator was disconnected as the right of privacy of an incompetent woman was allowed to overcome the state's interest in the conservation of human life. "The interest of the state weakens," said the *Quinlan* court, "and the right of the individual grows as the degree of bodily invasion increases and the prognosis dims."[24] Also in a New York case, Brother Fox, a Catholic priest in a vegetative state, had made it known before he became incompetent that he would not want to be maintained by a respirator. His right of self-determination was not subordinated to the state's interest in preserving life.[25]

But then came *Cruzan v. Harmon*.[26] In the case, the parents of Nancy Cruzan, a thirty-three-year-old patient in a persistent vegetative state, requested a court order to stop tube feedings. The Missouri Supreme Court ruled that the interest of the state in preserving life would be used to force the patient to be artificially maintained. In order to assert the state's interest, the Missouri court adopted a "clear and convincing" standard of proof in the proceedings brought by the patient's parents to terminate artificial feeding. This placed the burden of proof on them to show their daughter's intentions regarding stoppage. They could not do so and their request for termination was denied. The U.S. Supreme Court granted *certiorari* to review the case on the issue of whether the federal Constitution allowed Missouri's actions. This was the heart of the case. The majority found that the Constitution did not prevent Missouri from adopting the standard of "clear and convincing evidence" to advance its interest in preserving life and that this interest was unqualified and absolute.[27] The high court's holding is narrowly limited to Missouri, but it is alarming to supporters of patient's rights. It opens wide the legal door to any other state wishing to ape Missouri and to assert such an interest to prevent the parents of patients from protecting them and acting on their behalf and to deny patients what appear to be their wishes and rights to refuse treatment. As one respected authority on health law wrote: "The truth is, if the state of Missouri can inflict its will on Cruzan and her family, none of us are safe from states that wish to control our health care decisions and our death" (Annas, 1990:672).

To sum up, it can be said that although the interests of the state, especially that of preserving life, are strong, the right of a competent adult to refuse all medical treatment has generally outweighed these interests. Based on one or more of the individual's rights to self-determination, informed consent, privacy, liberty, or religious convictions, both the law and the medical community today support the right of an adult patient who is competent to decline treatment, including life-sustaining therapy. **Form 1.2.1** provides a refusal to be signed by such a patient who acknowledges that he or she has received relevant and essential information and the opportunity to ask questions but has decided to refuse specified medical treatment. A patient who has understood the information received and has the capacity to provide informed refusal is not legally required to supply reasons for a refusal of treatment. However, since a patient's refusal of treatment is generally motivated by the patient's personal, religious, or philosophical perspectives, a form might clarify the patient's decision by recording the patient's views. Since reasons for refusal may vary among patients, a form might leave a blank space to be completed with reasons cited by a patient, or offer a generalized reason most patients will find acceptable. As one possible general reason for refusal, **Form 1.2.1** offers the view that specified medical treatments are considered heavy spiritual, psychological, physical, or economic burdens. The form also releases medical personnel and hospital from consequences attendant upon the refusal.

The form is to be signed by two witnesses, one of whom is neither the spouse nor a blood relative of the patient. The form is to be signed also by the attending physician.

1.3 HOSPITAL POLICY AND PROCEDURES— REFUSAL OF TREATMENT BY PATIENTS WITH DECISION-MAKING CAPACITY AND WITHOUT DECISION-MAKING CAPACITY

A hospital policy and procedure should be developed and followed when proposed treatment is refused. **Form 1.3.1** suggests such a policy and procedure.

A policy of this kind addresses two situations: refusal by adult patients who are not terminal and not comatose and who have decision-making capacity; and refusal by their surrogates or proxies when decision-making capacity is absent. When treatment decisions for such patients are made by surrogates or proxies, the decisions are to be based on the subjective judgment standard and on their reasonable beliefs that the patient would have made the same decision. In the first situation, in the section "Procedure for a Patient with Decision-Making Capacity," the policy stipulates that the attending physician, in the presence of a witness, is to provide the patient with information pertinent to the patient's condition along with an explanation of the proposed intervention, possible alternatives, and their risks and benefits.

The policy provides for a witness to confirm the explanation and the patient's understanding of the information, appreciation of the situation, and ability to explain the reasons for refusal. The provision is used when the hospital wishes a nurse to attest to these circumstances in order to maintain a defense in any malpractice action based on the absence of informed consent brought against the hospital or physicians. If, however, a hospital believes that it may be better strategy that a nurse act only as a witness to the signature of a patient and that a physician alone be responsible for establishing the patient's informed consent, the provision should be omitted or limited to attesting only to the patient's signature.

The policy also states that the patient's decision-making capacity is to be evaluated. Normally, a patient is presumed to have the capacity to make health care decisions and give informed consent. The refusal of treatment by a patient with decision-making capacity will be respected, and a document stating the patient's refusal will be signed by the patient, witnessed, and signed by the attending physician. Such a document is provided in **Form 1.2.1**.

But if decision-making capacity is in doubt, the policy provides guidelines in the section "Procedure for a Patient Who Lacks Decision-Making Capacity" as to how and by whom the patient's capacity is to be evaluated. The attending physician should make the evaluation. If it is this physician's conclusion that capacity is lacking, a second physician also makes an evaluation. If the two physicians are in agreement that a patient lacks capacity to make health care decisions or give informed consent, the hospital is to enter both evaluations in the patient's medical record. This documentation establishes a rebuttable presumption that incapacity exists. In the real world of hospitals, however, where the mental incapacity of a patient is crystal clear to all interested parties, it is probable that, in spite of policy, the second opinion of a consulting physician will not be sought.

The policy also provides guidelines in the case of a patient without decision-making capacity. If a health care surrogate has been designated, notification is to be given to the surrogate that the surrogate's authority has begun. **Form 1.3.2** supplies such notification. If a surrogate has not been designated or is not available or willing to make health care decisions, an individual in a specified hierarchy of authority is to be selected as proxy to make them. The notification to the proxy is provided by **Form 1.3.3**. If the patient is an underage minor and not emancipated, a proxy is to be selected according to the following order: court-appointed guardian, parent, or nearest relative.

The attending physician is to provide a surrogate or proxy with an explanation that a witness is to attest. In an emergency life-threatening situation, however, if a surrogate or proxy is not able to act or is not available and there is substantial evidence of a patient's lack of capacity, a physician is authorized to override a patient's refusal of treatment. A surrogate's, guardian's, or proxy's refusal of treatment is a decision based on his or her reasonable belief that the refusal is a decision the patient would have made if capable of doing so. **Form 1.3.4** supplies the document to be signed by the surrogate, guardian, or proxy and witnessed.

If no one in the family circle can be located to act as proxy, guardianship proceedings will be necessary even though they may slow down or obstruct patient care or prevent critical care beds, always in short supply and costly, from being used for other patients. In some jurisdictions, it may take from one to four days to obtain a court appointment. A prudent hospital policy should anticipate and try to expedite such proceedings as soon as it becomes apparent to the hospital that no family member has been identified by a patient or that none may be available. **Form 1.3.1.1** provides an optional clause which might be added to a policy which calls for notice to be given to the hospital's social services department so that steps can be taken immediately to facilitate proceedings.

The refusal-of-treatment policies of some hospitals give no effect to refusal of medical treatment by a patient who is pregnant. For those hospitals wishing to adopt a similar policy, **Form 1.3.1.2** supplies an optional clause for insertion into the policy and into their refusal-of-treatment forms.

However, it will be noticed that **Form 1.3.1**, relating to the policy on refusal of treatment, and **Forms 1.1.4, 1.1.5,** and **1.2.1**, which permit patients, including Jehovah's Witnesses, to refuse treatment, are deliberately silent on the subject of pregnancy and clearly imply that a woman who is pregnant is permitted to refuse treatment that she does not want. The position taken by these forms is in deference to the decisions of the U.S. Supreme Court in *Cruzan* and judicial decisions on the state level that make it clear that every competent adult has the constitutional and common-law right to refuse treatment. The woman does not lose this right because she is pregnant, at least not prior to the viability of her fetus.

1.4 LIMITATION OF RIGHT OF REFUSAL OF LIFE-SUSTAINING TREATMENT TO TERMINALLY ILL PATIENTS

But is the right to refuse life-sustaining treatment limited to terminally ill patients? There is no logical or practical reason for such a limitation. Several court decisions involving patients who were not terminally ill and who might have lived for long periods if life supports had not been discontinued (including the one in *Brophy*, where the patient was not in a terminal condition) have recognized that all patients in this category have the same right as patients who are terminally ill to choose whether to accept or reject such treatment.[28] Meisel correctly labels as a "myth" the notion that a patient must be terminally ill before life support can be stopped (Meisel, 1991:1498).

1.5 DEPENDENCE OF RIGHT OF REFUSAL ON WHETHER CARE IS EXTRAORDINARY OR ORDINARY

Does the right to refuse depend on whether the care is extraordinary or ordinary? The earliest mention of "extraordinary means" of medical treatment can be found in Roman Catholic moral theology. While it held that human life is a precious and divine gift, it also taught that there is no ethical obligation to preserve it at all costs. It was not ethically obligatory to employ extraordinary means to prolong life if such treatment offered no hope of benefit to a patient and created psychological, economic, or spiritual burdens for the family (McCartney, 1990). Among ethicists and in the medical community, the distinction arose between "ordinary" life-sustaining treatment, which could not be ethically withheld or withdrawn from a patient, and "extraordinary" treatment, which could be. The *Quinlan* court and other courts took note of it. It is now recognized, however, by ethicists as well as the medical community and courts that the right to accept or refuse treatment is not dependent on the description of medical procedures as "ordinary" or "extraordinary" and "major" or "minor" because these are legally indistinguishable. It is a meaningless distinction because it is difficult to say just when care is extraordinary and when it is ordinary. So rapid have been advances in medical technology that what was extraordinary is now ordinary. Most important, whether treatment is extraordinary or ordinary, a competent adult has the right to decline both.[29]

1.6 TERMINATION OF LIFE-SUSTAINING TREATMENT ALREADY BEGUN

Does the right to refuse life-sustaining treatment extend to terminating treatment which has been started? The right to stop treatment is concomitant with the right to refuse it.[30] Stopping treatment understandably may cause the physician more emotional concern than not starting it because it is an act that may bring on death. While death may also come if treatment is not started, the difference is that it does so because of an omission, not an act. Nevertheless, if the patient has refused it, treatment must be withdrawn.

Like the distinction between ordinary and extraordinary treatment, any drawn between withholding and withdrawing treatment has no legal or moral significance. About the concern some physicians may have about greater legal liability for withdrawing treatment than for withholding it, the President's Commission for the Study of Ethical Problems said: "Nothing in law—certainly not in the context of the doctor-patient relationship—makes stopping treatment a more serious issue than not starting treatment. In fact, not starting treatment that might be in the patient's best interest is more likely to be held a civil or criminal wrong than stopping treatment which has proved unavailing" (President's Commission, 1983:77).

1.7 RIGHT OF REFUSAL OF LIFE-SUSTAINING TREATMENT AND ARTIFICIAL FEEDING

Does the right to refuse life-sustaining treatment also include the right to reject the artificial provision of nutrition and hydration? Life-sustaining treatment which may be refused includes chemotherapy, renal dialysis, mechanical ventilation, and antibiotics. The question of its extension to artificial procedures for the provision of hydration and nutrition to patients incapable of digesting, swallowing, or taking sustenance orally creates the disturbing prospect of withdrawing from a patient what some see as the basic necessity of life and has become the most hotly contested of all the questions so far considered. It arouses sharp divisions of opinion among philosophers, ethicists, and jurists. In *Brophy*, for example, two judges dissented from the majority opinion approving the removal of Brophy's gastrostomy tube, one of them saying that the withdrawal of the provision of food and water "is a particularly difficult, painful and gruesome death."[31] Reflecting this view, the living will statutes of some states distinguished artificial feeding from other medical treatment which could be refused. In recent years, however, one by one courts have begun to answer yes to the foregoing question. They held that the artificial provision of food and water was indistinguishable from other invasive forms of life-sustaining procedures, such as artificial breathing furnished by a respirator.[32] The American Medical Association (AMA) is in accord with these rulings. A statement of the AMA Council on Ethical and Judicial Affairs (1986), stated that "Life-prolonging treatment includes medication and artificially or technologically supplied respiration, nutrition, or hydration." In 1990, in *Cruzan v. Director, Missouri Department of Health*, the U.S. Supreme Court, making no distinction between artificial feeding and other medical treatment, added its authority to the proposition that the Constitution grants a competent adult the right to refuse life-sustaining hydration and nutrition.[33]

1.8 RIGHT OF REFUSAL OF MEDICAL TREATMENT AND EUTHANASIA

Does the right to refuse life-sustaining treatment extend to requesting and receiving euthanasia? Is there any real distinction, ask those who argue in favor of "aid-in-dying," between letting patients die at their request and killing them at their request? There is a legal distinction which prevents the right to refuse treatment from being enlarged to include the power to enlist the aid of doctors to kill. It is between passive euthanasia—withholding or withdrawing life-sustaining treatment at the request of a patient, which the law permits—and active euthanasia—the intentional act which causes death. Examples of active euthanasia include affirmatively acting to poison a patient by injecting large doses of morphine and injecting intravenously large doses of air. Even if such an act is done out of great love and kindness, the present common-law and state penal statutes condemn it as a crime, whether they treat it as murder or as aiding and abetting a suicide.

If patient autonomy is respected by the medical community and if competent adults have the right voluntarily to refuse every treatment option that might save their lives, why should physicians question honoring the wishes of suffering patients who ask them to end their lives humanely, swiftly, and painlessly by giving aid-in-dying? Because there is as well the ethical distinction between healing and killing. The physician-patient relationship is committed to healing and should not be converted from one in which the physician is to heal into one in which the physician kills. The prohibition against killing which can be traced back to Hippocrates provides an important basis for trust in the physician and the medical profession. Its removal would create irreparable harm (Beauchamp and Childress, 1989). Physicians have no moral obligation to accede to the request of a patient to use their medical expertise to terminate the life of the patient when doing so violates the medical code of ethics.

1.9 RIGHT OF REFUSAL AND INSTITUTIONAL POLICIES

Can the mission or policies of health care facilities override the right exercised by competent adults to refuse life-sustaining treatment? The right of competent adults to decline medical treatment may be recognized but what is the result when these rights clash with the philosophy of policies of a health care facility and its medical staff? Hospitals or nursing homes may refuse to carry out patients' wishes to decline life-sustaining treatment on the grounds that they contradict the institution's religious or moral convictions. Since these clashes seem to be on an inevitable collision course with the courts, it seems profitable to consider two related issues now and a third in section 1.10.

First, what can patients do to implement their rights and still avoid costly, vexatious, and time-consuming litigation? They can take the steps Patricia Brophy failed to take. *Brophy* is remarkable because it is a case that should never have been brought into the courtroom at all. In spite of all her reflections and discussions, Patricia Brophy did not do the obvious. She did not make use of the power she had to discharge the recalcitrant physicians who were unwilling to honor her wishes and to find others who were more understanding and supportive. She did not remove her husband from the uncooperative hospital to another facility in the state or out of state where her medical decision would be respected. Other doctors and institutions would not have been difficult to find because, as the high court noted in its decision, "a significant portion of the medical community disagrees with New England Mt. Sinai Hospital and considers it appropriate to withhold hydration and nutrition from individuals like Brophy."[34] The refusal of the hospital to do what other hospitals in Massachusetts were willing to do is a further factor that makes the entry of *Brophy* into the courts extraordinary.

Should patients decide to leave an institution whose philosophy or policy opposes their requests in order to seek out another and more sympathetic health facility, the institution cannot hold them against their will since that might expose the institution to liability for false imprisonment. To protect itself against claims that it abandoned or discharged a patient in need of medical treatment, the institution should ask the patient to sign a statement to the effect that the patient is leaving the hospital of his or her own free will and against its advice, that the patient has been advised of the dangers attendant on leaving, assumes all responsibility for the results of a premature departure, and releases the institution, the attending physician, and all others concerned with the care of the patient from all liability. **Form 1.9.1** provides these statements.

If a patient refuses to sign the statement, he or she cannot be confined in the facility until the statement is signed. The only course left to the institution in such a case is for the attending physician to document the situation on the medical record; the entry should be witnessed by the hospital staff having knowledge of the occurrence.

If, as in *Brophy*, the courts are called on to resolve the clash between patient and hospital, the discussion in section 1.2 relating to the ethics of the medical profession suggests that the interests of the patient should prevail. Thus, in *In re Jobes*,[35] where a permanently unconscious woman was sustained by a feeding tube, and in *In re Requena*,[36] where a patient with amyotrophic lateral sclerosis wished to reject artificial feeding, courts have concluded that a patient's right to refuse treatment cannot be abridged and transcends the policy of a health care facility. In *Bartling v. Superior Court*,[37] a hospital, described as "Christian, pro-life oriented," refused to disconnect a respirator in spite of the written requests of a seventy-year-old competent patient and his wife and, in fact, placed restraints on his wrists to prevent his attempts at removing the respirator himself. The court decided that, if the right of the patient was to be meaningful, "it must be paramount to the interests of the patient's hospital and doctors."

1.10 FORCING HEALTH PROVIDERS TO COMPLY WITH PATIENTS' WISHES

Can recalcitrant health care providers be required by a court to accede to a patient's wishes? If not, what is the alternative? It is not the facility that must actually attend and furnish treatment for a patient; it is the physicians and nurses in it who must. In most cases, no court should force them to provide treatment which violates their personal moral beliefs (President's Commission, 1982:48). The patient should be transferred to an alternative facility.

Indeed, in *Brophy*, the Supreme Judicial Court of Massachusetts did not compel New England Mt. Sinai Hospital to remove Brophy's gastrostomy tube. Rather, it authorized the hospital to transfer the patient to another facility. (He was, in fact, transferred to a hospital in Concord, where the tube was removed and he died.) But in some instances there can be no transfer because other facilities cannot be found willing to accept a patient in a permanently vegetative state and to honor the wishes of his family to remove his feeding tube.[38] Then, too, a patient may feel so close to the "familiar surroundings and the familiar people" in a hospital that it is "home" to her and she would be devastated by a transfer to different surroundings even in another hospital ready to admit her and honor her wish to stop life support.[39] In such cases some state courts have ordered private hospitals and nursing homes to comply with the patient's or family's wishes and to care for the patient until death. Publicly owned hospitals, as arms of the federal, state, or municipal governments that operate them, would not appear to be entitled to adopt religious or partisan policies that contravene a patient's rights.[40] Adverse state and federal court rulings such as these suggest that private and public health care institutions should seriously reconsider interfering with a patient's rights because of the philosophies and values of the institution.

1.11 TERMINATION OF LIFE SUPPORT AND COURT APPROVAL

Is the approval of a court necessary before life-sustaining treatment can be withdrawn or withheld? In 1977, in *Superintendent of Belchertown State School v. Saikewicz*,[41] the Supreme Judicial Court of Massachusetts made plain its view that the right forum for life-and-death decisions was the courts and nowhere else: "We take a dim view of any attempt to shift the ultimate decision making responsibility away from the duly established courts of proper jurisdiction to any committee, family or group, ad hoc or permanent. Thus, we reject the approach . . . of entrusting the decision whether to continue artificial life support to the patient's guardian, family, attending doctors, or hospital 'ethics committee.' "

In spite of this language, the general legal trend seems to accept that in the typical case, the decision to withhold or withdraw treatment by a competent patient, or by someone acting on behalf of a patient who does not have the capacity for making the decision, may be implemented without judicial approval. While some courts[42] have reconfirmed *Saikewicz*, a number of other courts have begun to recognize that they should not always intervene because it is more compassionate not to do so. In *In re Jobes*,[43] a nursing home rejected a distraught family's request to discontinue the tubal feeding of their thirty-two-year-old daughter who had been in a permanently unconscious state for seven years. In ordering stoppage of the feeding, the New Jersey Supreme Court said: "Courts are not the proper place to resolve the agonizing personal problems that underlie these cases. Our legal system cannot replace the more intimate struggle that must be borne by the patient, those caring for the patient, and those who care about the patient." In the *Quinlan* case, where the family was allowed to make treatment decisions for a daughter, further reasons were given for keeping life-and-death decisions out of the courts: "We consider that a practice of applying to a court to confirm said decisions would generally be inappropriate, not only because that would be a gratuitous encroachment upon the medical profession's field of competence, but because it would be impossibly cumbersome."[44] The recent *Cruzan* decision by the U.S. Supreme Court did not affect medical practice as to require prior court approval for termination of treatment decisions made in a private forum.

Nor is court approval necessary for the termination of life support when a patient lacks decision-making capacity and has left no advance directive. Local statutes may allow individuals in the following order of priority to be selected as proxies to make treatment decisions: the legal guardian, if one has been appointed previously; the patient's spouse; an adult child or, if there is more than one, the majority of adult children; a parent; an adult sibling; or an adult relative. In some states, decision making has been extended beyond the family circle to a close personal friend—someone of at least eighteen years of age who has shown care and concern for the patient and is familiar with the patient's beliefs. No court order is needed, and expensive and dilatory proceedings to appoint a legal guardian with authority to consent to medical treatment are avoided. It is a frequent occurrence in cases of patients without decision-making capacity who have left no advance directives, however, that none of the individuals who might serve as proxies are identified by the patient or, if identified, they cannot be found after diligent efforts. In such cases, guardianship proceedings cannot be avoided and must be instituted to appoint someone to make health care decisions.

Other situations may arise also when judicial intervention into the sphere of life-sustaining treatment may be required. Physicians or hospitals may fear legal liability or be unsure of the law if they terminate treatment for a patient, competent or incompetent. They may go to court as a prudent measure because they want legal protection or immunity before starting or stopping treatment. A judicial decision may also be requested by a hospital or physicians who challenge the decision of a surrogate. Under some statutes, judicial intervention can be sought by any person affected by the decision, such as the patient's family, the health care facility, or the attending physician. The grounds for review include the following: (1) the surrogate or proxy was not properly designated; (2) the designation of the surrogate is not effective any longer; (3) the decision is not in accord with the patient's known desires; (4) the patient's advance directive is ambiguous; or (5) the patient changed his or her mind after it was executed.[45]

2

Living Wills

2.1 ADVANCE DIRECTIVES

An *advance directive* permits competent adults, if they wish, to make prear-rangements for the health care to be given them in the future. One rationale for the advance directive is that if adults with decision-making capacity can personally accept or refuse medical or surgical treatment, there should be no legal or other reason why they should not be able to accept or refuse it through a directive or even through an agent in advance of the loss of such capacity. Another rationale is that we have the right to exercise and retain control over decisions about our health care. The advance directive furnishes a vehicle by which adults, with the ability to make choices and decisions concerning the provision, withholding, or withdrawing of medical treatment, give oral or written directions to physicians to control treatment in the future when decision-making capacity may be absent, or by which adults may designate someone to make treatment decisions for them if they do not have the capacity to make and communicate such decisions.

2.2 LIVING WILL STATUTES: COMMON PROVISIONS

There are several types of advance directives. The type most commonly thought of is the *living will* also known as a *declaration*. The case of Karen Ann Quinlan made famous the plight of the patient in a persistent vegetative state who could not exercise any decision-making powers. Motivated by her case, California passed the first living will statute in

1976. Since then, possibly motivated as well by the confusing number and
variety of grounds and arguments provided by the courts for upholding
the right to refuse treatment, forty-five states, the District of Columbia,
and two U.S. territories, Puerto Rico and Guam, have also enacted such
statutes. There are differences among the statutes but they all appear to
share the following important provisions.

Terminal Condition

Any competent adult may make a living will or declaration that directs
physicians what to do or not to do in the future if that person is terminally
ill. The uniform intent of all statutes is to attach this condition to all living
wills. The declaration does not become effective or controlling until the
individual is diagnosed as suffering from a terminal condition.

A *terminal condition* generally means a condition caused by injury, disease,
or illness from which there is no reasonable probability of recovery and which,
without treatment, can be expected to cause death. Some forward-looking
statutes have expanded this definition to include a persistent vegetative state,[46]
a permanent and irreversible condition of unconsciousness in which there is
an absence of voluntary action or cognitive behavior of any kind and an
inability to communicate or interact purposefully with the environment. The
only variation among the statutes is with respect to the diagnosis, as some
statutes require that only the attending or treating physician is to determine
that a terminal condition exists, while other statutes require that the attending
or treating physician and a consulting physician must determine that there is
no medical probability of the patient's recovery from his or her condition.
The statutes, however, do not require the existence of a terminal condition
at the time the declaration is made. The declaration is for people looking
ahead and who want to participate in decisions about their treatment in the
event they have a terminal condition.

Immunity from Liability

A health care facility, physician, or anyone under the physician's direction
is guaranteed immunity from criminal prosecution, civil liability, or discipli-
nary measures for unprofessional conduct for carrying out the wishes expressed in a living will by a patient with a terminal condition. The guarantee
is ineffective if good faith on the part of the person effectuating these wishes
does not exist. The probability of showing failure to act in good faith "beyond
a reasonable doubt" in a criminal case or by a preponderance of the evidence
in a civil suit, however, is highly remote.

Conflict Between Patients' Rights and Medical Policies or Ethics

Living will statutes of most states have tried to resolve the difficult problem noted above of the conflict between the rights of patients to refuse life-sustaining treatment and the policies of health care facilities or the personal beliefs of health professionals which prevent them from carrying out the patient's requests. The legislation in many states provides that if, because of moral beliefs, a health provider will not comply with a living will, the provider must make reasonable efforts to transfer the patient to another provider who will comply with the living will, if, at the time of admission, the patient was informed of the policies of the provider concerning such beliefs and if the patient is not in an emergency condition. The costs of the transfer will be borne by the provider. If the patient is not transferred, the wishes of the patient will be honored.

Declarations Executed in Other States

Living wills executed and valid in another state are recognized as valid.

Life Insurance

Life insurance policies are to be unaffected by a living will.

Suicide, Euthanasia, and Homicide

The making of a living will does not constitute suicide, euthanasia, or homicide.

2.3 LIVING WILLS: FORM, CONTENT, AND PROCEDURES

A living will may be either a written document whose execution meets the strict requirements for the execution of a formal will, or an oral statement that is witnessed. Thus, in some states, if the person is not, for physical reasons, able to sign the declaration, an oral one may be made, but then one of the witnesses must sign the person's name to a written declaration in the person's presence and at the person's direction.

The person making the living will has the responsibility of notifying the attending physician that a living will has been made. However, if the maker of the living will is physically incapacitated when admitted to a health care facility, someone else is to give notice to the attending physician or facility of the living will's existence. On notification, the physician or facility must make the living will part of the medical record.

Artificial feeding was something several courts and state legislatures were reluctant to accept as distinguishable from other medical procedures that could be declined. Some judicial decisions and statutes had flatly decreed that it was required to provide comfort care and was not included in the life-sustaining procedure that might be withheld or withdrawn.[47] In other states, another statutory provision was enacted to the effect that artificial feeding would be excluded from this procedure unless a person gave specific directions in a living will that it be withheld or withdrawn.[48] Even though these directions might be given, however, some statutes also authorized the patient's family to overrule a declarant's wish in spite of the fact that it had been expressed in a living will[49]—in effect, what had been given to the declarant could hardly be called a right to refuse artificial feeding because it was subject to the family's veto. With the *Cruzan* ruling by the U.S. Supreme Court that a competent adult had the constitutional right to refuse life-sustaining therapy including artificially supplied nutrition and hydration, and in view of common-law rights recognized by state courts to reject treatment, these kinds of statutes appear to burden or restrain these rights too much, and their constitutionality is in grave doubt.

All state statutes suggest a form of declaration that, with little variation, is also suggested by virtually every other living will statute. In some states, a declaration must substantially follow the statutory form; in others a form of living will is only suggested. If a form need not be in the form prescribed by a statute, people should design their own. A living will should be tailor-made to suit and express the wishes and needs of the individual. Since living wills vary with the individual, they need not contain identical provisions. The documents and clauses suggested here offer patients some options from which to choose.

With the Patient Self-Determination Act, to be discussed later, Congress sought to widen public understanding about advance directives. To help with the education process, **Form 2.3.1**, which answers some of the frequently asked questions about living wills, might be used in physicians' offices or hospitals.

Form 2.3.2 offers a basic living will declaration which may be used where a local statute allows only the attending physician to determine if a person has a terminal condition. **Form 2.3.3** may be used where two physicians are required by statute to determine that a condition is hopeless. Whatever form is used to establish a terminal condition, the living will becomes effective not only when such a condition exists, but also only when the declarant is incapable of providing informed consent. While he or she has decision-making capacity, treatment can be discussed with a physician and decisions made.

These forms will suffice in jurisdictions which have always included artificial feeding in life-sustaining procedures that may be refused in a living will and in those that have repealed their living will statutes which had excluded artificial feeding from these life-sustaining procedures. In states, however, where artificial feeding may not be withheld or withdrawn in the absence of a specific direction expressed in a living will, **Form 2.3.4** provides a clause which may be used to express the declarant's wish either to withhold or withdraw or not to withhold or withdraw such feeding.

The second paragraph in all forms contains general statements instructing a physician not to prolong the patient's dying. If nothing more is said, this statement will apply. When the living will gets into a hospital ward, however, health care personnel may find it vague or ambiguous, and each physician or health care facility may interpret it differently. This kind of ambiguity should be avoided. It may allow some physicians to reject a living will, or it may force physicians to take time to reach an agreement with the patient's family about the patient's true wishes. Meanwhile, the patient's pain and suffering may be prolonged while the costs of care rise dramatically. A prudent declarant should consider completing the "Additional Directions" section above the line on which the declarant's signature appears. This is shown on **Form 2.3.5**. It will allow the declarant to specify any procedures or treatments that are not wanted, such as cardiopulmonary resuscitation, kidney dialysis, mechanical respiration, major surgery, chemotherapy or radiation, invasive diagnostic tests, intravenous therapy, antibiotics, or tubal feeding. The declarant's wishes regarding these procedures or treatments should have been clarified by discussions with his or her physicians about the kinds of procedures or treatments that are most often used when illness is severe and recovery unlikely and the kinds relevant to the declarant's condition that might be used. The section might also contain requests such as being sent from the hospital to the declarant's home to die. If a declarant is anxious about pain control, a statement such as the following might be added: "I want to receive as much pain medication as necessary to ensure my comfort even if it means hastening my death."

As an alternative to **Forms 2.3.2** and **2.3.3**, Emanuel and Emanuel (1989) have developed a form of medical directive which sets forth four illness scenarios. Patients indicate in each of them their choices concerning various kinds of life-support procedures or treatments such as those suggested in the preceding paragraph.

Some living will statutes provide that if the individual making the declaration is a pregnant female, the living will is not effective during the pregnancy. To comply with such statutes, a clause to be inserted in the living will has been shown in **Form 2.3.6.** If a female has made a living will, designated a surrogate, and is pregnant, other living will statutes do not permit the surrogate to consent to withholding or withdrawing life-sustaining treatment for the pregnant patient prior to viability unless the living will has delegated this authority. **Form 2.3.7** contains a clause that permits an individual to confer or refuse to confer such authority

Each state has a statutory form of living will. These forms should be sufficient to permit an individual to complete it. It need not be prepared by an attorney unless there is a question about the legal import of the document. Individuals can select among the various clauses offered here. Those desired can be commingled in the basic form, those found to be unsuitable can be omitted, or other clauses can be substituted. When a person finally selects a form, it should be dated and signed by the patient in the presence of two adult witnesses, neither of whom is a spouse or a blood relative of the patient or a surrogate designated by the patient to make health care decisions. The witnesses should subscribe the will. Since patients may request a health provider to witness a declaration, it should be noted that while some statutes may preclude a provider or its employees from serving as a health care surrogate, no statute disqualifies a health professional from being a witness to a declaration. In the event that the patient is physically unable to sign the living will, a witness should sign the patient's name in the presence of the patient and at the patient's direction. The living will statutes do not require the living will to be notarized.

A living will can be revoked at any time. Several methods are authorized by the statutes. It can be physically destroyed or cancelled by the declarant or by someone who does so at the direction and in the presence of the declarant. The declarant can sign and date a written revocation, such as is suggested in **Form 2.3.8**, or make an oral statement expressing the intention to revoke. Should the declarant later execute a living will materially different from the previous one, this act would constitute a revocation. Whichever method of revocation is adopted, in order to be effective it must be communicated to the attending physician, the health care facility, and the person designated as surrogate.

If the living will is not revoked, it should be reviewed periodically to be sure that it has kept up with changing laws. A document made a considerable time before it is needed may raise questions about how well and truly it reflects the present intentions of a declarant now unable to express his or her wishes. Redating and reinitialing it from time to time, however, will help avoid this problem as it will suggest that the old living will is still current.

Surveys show that the great majority of doctors support the living will (Orentlicher, 1990; Zinber, 1989). But why should patients make one? The case of Nancy Cruzan helps provide an answer.

After an automobile accident in 1983, Nancy Cruzan was taken to the Mt. Vernon State Hospital in Missouri. She suffered permanent brain damage and went into a coma and a persistent vegetative state. Cruzan was kept alive by nutrition and hydration delivered through a gastrostomy tube implanted by surgeons in her stomach; the tube might prolong her life for another fifteen to thirty years. A year before the automobile accident, she told a roommate that she "didn't want to live" as a "vegetable" and that if she "couldn't do things for herself even halfway, let alone not at all, she would not want to live that way and she hoped that her parents would know that." Her father and mother, convinced that their daughter would not want to live in her present condition, tried to exercise her right to decline life support and asked that it be stopped. But the Missouri Supreme Court discarded Nancy Cruzan's statements made before her incompetence on the ground that they were unreliable. It insisted on "clear and convincing" evidence of her wishes; these statements, it said, were not such evidence and Missouri would force her to be kept alive.[50] When the case came before the U.S. Supreme Court, the high court found that Missouri's strict evidential standard of clear and convincing evidence did not conflict with the Constitution and that its requirement could be imposed in order to prevent a death decision and advance the state's interest in preserving life.[51] The requirement imposed by Missouri is not unusual. Other state courts have also ruled that before life support can be stopped there must be clear and convincing proof articulating a patient's wish to terminate treatment.

The U.S. Supreme Court's decision has no application to patients with decision-making capacity or to those who lack it but, prior to incompetency, left clear evidence of their desires. But it does apply in cases where patients have given no advance directions and cannot be judged as having decision-making capacity. The decision serves notice that the common-law and constitutional right to refuse treatment, while granted to all, will be exercisable by surrogates only in the few cases of those willing to think about dying and death who have had the foresight to leave clear and specific directions spelling out their intentions about being allowed to die.

Other cases also serve notice that when no such directions are left behind and courts, families, and medical personnel struggle to arrive at an understanding of the patient's true wishes, a case may take days, weeks, months, or years before it is decided in the judicial forum. In consequence, the dying processes and sufferings of patients are prolonged to that extent, and they often die still undergoing unwanted treatment before a court decision is finally made in their cases. Of the many tragic examples of this kind is the case of Brother Fox, a Catholic priest who, during discussions with the staff at the Catholic school where he lived, had orally expressed his objection to the use of any extraordinary care to sustain him if he were ever in a vegetative condition. He was placed on a respirator after an operation in October 1979 precipitated him into a persistent vegetative state. He was still on it and finally died in January 1980 while the courts were still considering whether the evidence showed clearly his desire not to have his life extended by life-sustaining treatment. In March 1981, the New York Court of Appeals held that the evidence was clear and convincing of his wish to discontinue the treatment.[52]

The significance of *Cruzan* is that we must anticipate our possible incapacity to participate in treatment decisions in the future and leave living wills, or else run the risk of having the state intervene to take from us control of our own lives and from our families control of the lives of those closest to them. A state like Missouri might impose a strict standard of persuasion concerning our wishes in order to promote its interest and might require clear and convincing evidence of our wishes before stopping life support that sustains us as objects of medical technology. Without a living will directing such stoppage, an undue burden is placed on those trying to have an incapable patient's treatment stopped. On the other hand, a living will would meet a state's test of a clear and convincing demonstration of the wishes of a terminally ill patient to stop treatment. Many statutes expressly provide that a living will establishes a rebuttable presumption of clear and convincing evidence of these wishes.

In *Cruzan*, the Missouri Supreme Court[53] showed another dimension of state interference made possible by the absence of a living will. Courts have long recognized as surrogate decision makers close members of the family and have accorded them the right to make treatment decisions for incompetent family members.[54] The assumption is that parents will act in the best interests of their children.[55] The medical community also has traditionally recognized that the family is best qualified to make substituted medical judgment for an incompetent loved one. This recognition is shared by the President's Commission for the Study of Ethical Problems (1983) and the Hastings Center (1987). In view of this medical practice and recognition, the Missouri state court's decision in *Cruzan*, to which the authority of the U.S. Supreme Court was added, shocked many by rejecting the decision of loving and caring parents to withdraw artificial hydration and nutrition from their daughter. Thus a state, to promote its interest in preserving life, may intervene to dislodge the family as decision makers and replace them with strangers and state agents who are unfamiliar with a patient's wishes and values and will force continued treatment of a patient when there is no clear and convincing evidence of the patient's wishes expressed before incompetency to terminate the treatment. This, said Cruzan's attorney, exemplifies "the most offensive kind of state interference in our private lives" (Colby, 1990:6).

The lesson of *Cruzan* is that we had better become informed about and prepare living wills if we want to prevent ourselves and our families from experiencing what happened to Nancy Cruzan and her parents. Living wills ensure that treatment decisions can be made intelligently for us and that they are in line with our wishes expressed before mental and physical incapacities deprive us of decision-making powers.

3

Surrogate Decision Making

3.1 DECISION-MAKING CAPACITY AND THE RIGHT TO REFUSE TREATMENT

The doctrine of informed consent requires that a patient has the mental capacity to understand the medical information provided by the physician, to weigh the benefits and risks of the treatment or procedure proposed and of alternative therapies, and to make rational judgments to accept or decline the proposed course of action. The right to refuse life-sustaining treatment is, therefore, interwoven with such capacity.

The terms *competence* and *decision-making capacity* are used in reference to the question of whether the capacity exists. But *competence* is a legal term of interest to the courts who make rulings about it and appoint legal guardians for those adjudicated to be incapable of taking care of their persons or personal or financial affairs. In the medical world, where the concern is more narrowly limited to whether a patient has the ability to make a special medical decision as distinguished from the ability to decide to sell real property or the knowledge of how to manage a business, the legal standard is not used. There "competence" becomes "decision-making capacity" (Council on Ethical and Judicial Affairs, 1992). Competence "can be restated in the medical care context by saying that if an individual understands and appreciates the information needed to give informed consent, then that individual is competent to give both informed consent and to refuse consent" (Annas and Glantz, 1986:118) to a treatment option. Normally, a patient will be presumed to have the physical and mental ability to make and communicate decisions to give or refuse informed consent and they will be honored. Of course, the patient will have consulted with the attending physician and may wish to consult as well with family, friends, lawyers, and clergy. But the final decision rests with only the patient.

When might doubt arise concerning the patient's capacity to make health care decisions? If a patient is in accord with a proposed course of action, it is unlikely that a physician will question the patient's capacity. It is when a patient is uncooperative and refuses that capacity may be in issue, although, from the legal perspective, patients are entitled to be unwise or foolish or wrong in the doctor's view and still not necessarily be lacking in decision-making capacity. A legitimate example of when the question of capacity for taking part in end-of-life decisions would arise might be in the cases of patients in an intensive care unit. They may lack decision-making capacity because they may be encephalopathic as a result of sepsis, hypoxia, or liver disease.

The attending physician, who knows the patient and the patient's medical situation best, has the primary responsibility for evaluating decision-making capacity. The medical literature suggests various tests which may be used to help physicians assess the existence or nonexistence of the capacity (Kutner, Ruark, and Raffin, 1991; Applebaum and Grisso, 1988). Generally, they boil down to whether a patient has the physical or mental ability to understand information pertaining to his or her physical condition, appreciate the meaning of the information and its consequences, manipulate the information rationally, and then express and communicate a knowing and willful decision.

It is sometimes asserted that "Competent patients have the right to decide whether to accept or reject proposed medical care. Patients thought to be incompetent are denied this right" (Applebaum and Grisso, 1988:1635). If statements such as these are interpreted literally, they are wrong and misleading because almost every state court has recognized that the common-law and constitutional right to refuse medical treatment does not depend on, and is not denied because of, the quality of a patient's life. Whether the incompetent patient is an elderly one whose physical and mental functions are severely impaired,[56] a profoundly retarded one,[57] or one in a persistent vegetative state,[58] courts recognize that the same right to refuse treatment extends to all because the "value of human dignity" extends to all.[59] And this makes sense. In a country where fundamental rights are supposed to be guaranteed and protected, it is essential to protect them for all, especially for the mentally incompetent who no longer have or never had the ability to assert these rights themselves. Although *Cruzan* permitted a state to require clear and convincing evidence that a patient wished termination of her treatment, implicated in the ruling was the most recent recognition by the U.S. Supreme Court that the right of Nancy Cruzan to refuse medical treatment was not diminished because she had become incompetent.

But if physically or mentally incapacitated people leave no advance directives prior to incompetency and now do not have the ability to make conscious choices and personally and directly to express their choices to refuse life-sustaining treatment, they are denied the ability to exercise their right to refuse treatment. If the above quoted statement is interpreted in this way, it is correct. The right exists, but how can they exercise it? This is the real question.

3.2 MECHANISMS FOR HEALTH CARE DECISION MAKING: HEALTH CARE SURROGATE, DURABLE POWER OF ATTORNEY FOR HEALTH CARE, AND PROXY

The only way to prevent this right from being lost or destroyed is to delegate the right to health care decision makers who will act for incompetent patients and exercise their rights of refusal. Decision makers designated by patients prior to incompetency are surrogates, people such as family members or close friends who are trusted to make decisions for patients when they cannot speak for themselves and who understand the wishes of the patients. It is especially important that surrogates know if a patient wishes treatment continued as long as it can be effective; if a patient does not want treatment started; or if it is started, when a patient would want it to be stopped. Surrogates should be willing to accept the responsibility imposed on them. Patients should make sure that their surrogates agree to act in accordance with their instructions.

The majority opinion in the U.S. Supreme Court's decision in *Cruzan* did not address specifically the issue of whether a state must give effect to surrogate decision making on behalf of patients, such as Nancy Cruzan, who have made no living wills and who are incapable of exercising the right to terminate life-sustaining treatment. The concurring opinion of Justice Sandra Day O'Connor did, however. "I also write separately," she said, "to emphasize that . . . [i]n my view, a duty may well be constitutionally required to protect the patient's liberty interest in refusing medical treatment." Her opinion that a constitutional guaranty would apply to treatment decisions made by an individual selected by a competent adult to do so had an effect on state legislatures. They initiated or amended legislation regarding several devices to permit surrogate decisions and with them a second generation of advance directives to succeed the living will that offer patients an assortment of prearrangements to meet their desires and needs regarding future medical treatment. For further ammunition in the educational campaign to increase public awareness about the types of advance directives and other matters relating to them, Form 3.2.1 responds to questions commonly asked by patients.

At least one weakness in the living will may have also prompted the creation of these devices. Although there is general recognition of the right of all individuals to make medical directives which are binding on physicians and although physicians are granted immunity from civil or criminal liability for carrying them out, living wills have not always proved effective. One study, for example, showed that medical care was not consistent with the previously expressed wishes of a declarant in twenty-four out of ninety-six cases (Danis et al., 1991). Although the study was confined to a nursing home, it seems to reflect a widespread grievance that living wills are frequently ignored. They can be ignored because living will statutes do not make it mandatory for physicians, health care facilities, or skilled-nursing facilities to honor living wills. Physicians often are reluctant to carry out instructions in a living will because they don't want problems with vociferous relatives who oppose the instructions. On the other hand, with the enactment of mechanisms for surrogate decision making, it is far less easy to ignore a flesh-and-blood person acting as the appointed representative of a patient and speaking with and giving instructions to the physician or facility from the perspective and with the voice of the patient.

One of the devices is provided by living will statutes which permit the designation of a surrogate to make treatment decisions if the patient cannot participate in a medical decision. The patient also must have been diagnosed as terminal to make the living will and the surrogate's authority effective. The clause in Form 3.2.2 permits this designation to be made in a living will. Making a designation is optional and failure to make the designation will not invalidate the living will. Patients should, however, consider filling in the designation clause in the form and authorizing a surrogate to make medical decisions for them when they cannot speak for themselves. The designation is not only a highly practical way that people can make sure that their wishes will be honored; the surrogate can make decisions in medical situations and for medical conditions or medical interventions patients could not foresee and can make these decisions in line with what the patients want. If the designated surrogate is the spouse of the declarant and subsequent to the designation their marriage should be annulled or dissolved, some statutes provide that the annulment or dissolution shall operate to revoke the designation unless the living will provides otherwise.

Guardianship procedures exist in all states. They permit a voluntary petition to be made to a court for a limited guardian who will exercise the powers that are specified by the court to care for the rights and persons of adults for whom the guardian is appointed. As a less expensive and restrictive alternative to these procedures, and as a way to protect the rights of patients from being lost because of physical or mental incapacity, another type of advance directive was created to implement surrogate decision making: the written designation by a principal of a health care surrogate who will make health care decisions in the event of the principal's incapacity to make such decisions. **Form 3.2.3** is provided as an advisory for patients wishing to be informed about a health care surrogate designation. The health care surrogate designation has a distinct advantage over the living will since it allows the surrogate to act whenever the principal is incapable of making medical decisions, not only when a terminal condition exists but at any other time when the principal may be seriously ill and not capable of speaking for himself or herself.

The principal must be a competent adult. The document may specify a time of termination, and if not, it remains in effect until revoked. It is to be signed by the principal or contain a signature acknowledged by the principal generally in the presence of two adult witnesses, neither of whom is to be the individual designated as health care surrogate and one of whom is not to be the spouse or blood relative of the principal. If the principal is not capable of signing the document, with the witnesses present, he or she may direct someone else to sign the principal's name. An alternate surrogate may also be designated to act if the original surrogate will not or cannot perform his or her duties. The principal must provide a copy of the instrument to the surrogate and should also provide copies to all those who may be concerned about the principal's health. Since there may be restrictions placed on who can serve as a surrogate—for example, the principal's health care providers and their employees and relatives, or the operators or employees of health care facilities in which patients reside or relatives of an operator or employee, may be precluded by some statutes—these laws should be consulted before a designation is made.

A form to designate a health care surrogate and an alternate surrogate is provided in **Form 3.2.4**. Alternate designations of health care surrogates can be used. One containing instructions concerning the witholding or withdrawing of life-sustaining procedures is provided in **Form 3.2.4.1**. For the patient who prefers a terse designation, **Form 3.2.4.2** is suggested.

The authority of a health care surrogate begins as soon as a principal is determined to be lacking the capacity to make health care decisions or provide informed consent. It continues until it is determined that the principal has regained capacity. The capacity of a patient should be assessed periodically to determine if it has been regained. Unless limited by the principal or by a state statute, the surrogate's authority is generally broad. The surrogate may make the decision to withhold or withdraw life-sustaining procedures. The surrogate's authority also extends to making all health care decisions for the principal in consultation with health care providers, the decisions to be in accordance with instructions given by the principal and in line with decisions the principal would have made under the circumstances if the principal had decision-making capacity; having access to the principal's clinical records; applying for all Medicare and Medicaid or other public benefits to which the principal may be entitled and, if needed to make an application for them; having access to the principal's assets, income, and financial and banking records to the extent required to make application; and authorizing the transfer from and admission to a health care facility.

As in the case of a living will, the dissolution or annulment of the marriage of the principal revokes the designation of the principal's former spouse as health care surrogate. Revocation can be prevented, however, by a contrary provision either in the health care designation or in the court order dissolving or annulling the marriage.

Unless a principal has specifically delegated written authority to a surrogate or unless the surrogate has obtained judicial approval, some statutes may restrict the authority of the health care surrogate and prevent him or her from consenting to abortion, sterilization, electroshock therapy, psychosurgery, experimental treatment or therapies not recommended by a federally approved institutional review board, voluntary admission to a mental health facility, or the withholding or withdrawing of life-sustaining treatment from a pregnant patient prior to viability of the fetus. If they become or are pregnant, women who wish to grant authority to their surrogates to withdraw or withhold life-sustaining procedures prior to the viability of their fetuses may specify their wishes in the "Additional Instructions" section of **Form 3.2.4**, using for example, the directions suggested by **Form 2.3.7**.

The durable power of attorney for health care constitutes a further mechanism for surrogate decision making. All states have durable power of attorney statutes. A durable power of attorney should be in writing, should state the relationship of the parties, and should be signed by an individual (the principal) and witnessed generally by two people, one of whom may not be the spouse or blood relative of the principal. It does not need to be notarized, although most forms contain space anyway for a notary public's acknowledgment of the execution of the instrument.

A power of attorney permits a principal to designate a person as attorney-in-fact on whom is conferred full and general powers to act for the principal with respect to the principal's real or personal property and business or private affairs.

In addition to these general powers, it should have been possible to use the durable power of attorney to authorize an attorney-in-fact to perform any act not specifically prohibited by statutes, including consenting to or refusing medical treatment (Collin et al., 1984). In 1987, the question was presented to an appellate court for the first time in the case of a woman who had used a power of attorney to empower an attorney-in-fact to make treatment decisions for her. The New Jersey Supreme Court ruled that although the state's durable power of attorney statute did not specifically authorize medical decisions to be made by an attorney-in-fact, the statute should be interpreted to allow such decisions to be made.[60] In view of this judicial view of durable power of attorney legislation, more legislation seemed redundant (Annas, 1991). Nevertheless, a movement can be observed toward further legislation as twenty-nine states and the District of Columbia passed or amended statutes specifically to provide for the creation of a durable power of attorney for health care that allows the designation of an attorney-in-fact to make treatment decisions. As with the designation of a health care surrogate, some statutes do not permit the appointment of a health care provider treating the principal, an employee or relative of the provider, the operator of a health care facility in which the principal resides, or an employee or relative of the operator. The appointment of an attorney-in-fact with only the authority to perform health care acts is suggested by **Form 3.2.5.** Like the health care surrogate designation, the durable power of attorney for health care is effective in nonterminal situations when the principal is unable to make medical decisions. But for those who wish to confer broad powers, alternative **Form 3.2.5.1** contains a durable power of attorney for health care which confers both general powers and the authority to make treatment decisions.

But there are differences among the provisions of the various durable power of attorney statutes. By way of illustration, the statutes of California and Rhode Island provide that attorneys-in-fact may consent to or refuse medical treatment, including withdrawing or withholding life-sustaining treatment. On the other hand, while the statutes of Colorado, Florida, North Carolina, and Pennsylvania empower attorneys-in-fact to make decisions and consent to medical procedures, they do not expressly permit the attorney-in-fact to withdraw consent or refuse them. **Form 3.2.5.1** reflects these restrictive laws. These statutes, however, may create controversies over a principal's wishes concerning refusing, withdrawing, or withholding life-sustaining treatment. They seem to mandate that the durable power of attorney cannot be used to refuse such treatment and that the only authority for and means of doing so is the living will. It seems important, however, that an attorney-in-fact be permitted to make all treatment decisions—not merely to consent but as well to withdraw consent and decline care and treatment if that is the principal's wish—and that the power of attorney expressly confers this authority. **Form 3.2.5**, following the California and Rhode Island statutes but not the others, clearly documents the principal's intentions in this respect.

Under the common law, an ordinary power of attorney remained effective until the principal died or revoked it. Similarly, the durable power of attorney remains valid until death or revocation unless the document states a time of termination. Both **Forms 3.2.5** and **3.2.5.1** contain clauses to this effect. Some statutes, however, provide that it will terminate after the lapse of a certain number of years but when this period expires, if the principal is unable to make health care decisions, the durable power of attorney will continue until the principal regains that ability.

What is the impact on these instruments of the incompetency of the principal? The common-law rule is that ordinary powers of attorney cease on the later mental incapacity of the principal.[61] It is just at the crucial moment when principals are incapable of speaking for themselves and need someone who knows their wishes to speak for them that the authority of the attorney-in-fact to speak is revoked and the ordinary power of attorney becomes useless.

It is here that the durable power of attorney steps into the breach in one of two ways. Under some statutes, a "springing" durable power of attorney will become effective on the incapacity of the principal. **Form 3.2.5** is in this category. But how is it to be determined that the principal has become incapable? This form contemplates a determination by a court. Is it always necessary to institute a court proceeding? An optional clause might be inserted in a durable power of attorney to avoid formal judicial intervention by making the incapacity of a principal a fact to be established by people in whom the principal has confidence. **Form 3.2.5.2** names the principal's spouse and lawyer as the individuals who will determine the principal's lack of capacity to manage the principal's affairs. **Form 3.2.5.3** nominates two doctors who will certify the principal's lack of decision-making capacity. **Form 3.4.1** might be used in part to certify their assessment of the principal's capacity. The statutes generally require the durable power of attorney to include specific wording, such as "This durable power of attorney shall not be affected by the disability of the principal." **Forms 3.2.5** and **3.2.5.1** contain this provision.

Patients who prepare advance directives should understand that the law does not prevent the use of all kinds—the living will, the health care surrogate designation, and the durable power of attorney—as supplementary to one another to give maximum protection in all medical situations. They should also be educated concerning the disposition to be made of their documents. Copies should go to anyone who will be aware that they are very sick. A living will should be given to their physicians. A health care surrogate designation and durable power of attorney for health care should go to the individuals they have appointed and with whom they have talked over their wishes. Other copies might also be given to their families, attorneys, ministers, priests, or rabbis. When they are admitted to a hospital, copies of their advance directives should also be provided to the hospital administration. It is also wise for them to carry in their wallets or purses next to their driver's licenses or health insurance cards, or to store in the glove compartment of their cars, another card describing where their advance directives can be found and the names, addresses, and telephone numbers of their surrogates. **Form 3.2.6** offers such a card.

If a patient who lacks or is impaired in decision-making capacity has made no advance directive and has appointed no surrogate, who makes health care decisions for the patient? In the past, the medical community has traditionally recognized close family members as health care decision makers despite an absence of express written or oral appointment by the patient. Who except the family that knows the patient best should be in a position to make decisions? Although the *Cruzan* case undermined the general medical practice of accepting family treatment decisions by its refusal to allow the patient's parents to speak for their daughter, the high courts of the states generally have supported the practice. In *Brophy* and *Quinlan*, for example, the courts confirmed it by granting letters of guardianship to a wife and father, respectively, to exercise the rights of the incompetent patients in those cases although the patients had never designated them. Many statutes provide another confirmatory device: the proxy, generally a family member who has not been previously expressly designated by a patient to make health care decisions but is authorized by statute to do so if a patient has not executed any advance directive appointing a surrogate or if a designated surrogate is not willing or able to carry out the surrogate's responsibilities. To avoid the risk of a state like Missouri becoming involved when no living will has been made and playing the role of decision maker in place of family members, many states have adopted proxy procedures that list potential proxies who will be given authority to decide for a patient in an order of priority described in Section 1.11. These statutes ensure that if there is no court-appointed guardian, members of the patient's family or sometimes a close personal friend will be authorized to make medical treatment decisions for incompetent patients. By virtue of these statutes, health care decisions will be made not by the state but by a proxy. If an appointed surrogate and an alternate surrogate (if there is one) are unwilling or unable to perform their duties, some statutes authorize a health care facility to fall back on the proxy device and seek the appointment of a legal guardian, someone within the family or a close friend, to take on the task.

3.3 HOSPITAL POLICY AND PROCEDURES—PATIENTS WITH ADVANCE DIRECTIVES

Form 3.3.1 contains a hospital policy dealing with advance directives, which are defined as a living will, a durable power of attorney, and a health care surrogate designation. It provides the procedures to be followed for each of these directives.

Generally, the procedures deal with what is required for the validity of living wills, whether written or oral, for notification of their existence to be given to the attending physician, for their documentation in the patient's medical record, and for revocation of the declarations.

The durable power of attorney should also be reviewed. Is it in writing? Is it signed by the principal and at least one witness? Does it contain the language required by all statutes to prevent it from ceasing on the incapacity of the principal? To ascertain if the durable power of attorney is still valid and the attorney-in-fact can still act under it, the hospital staff should make inquiries concerning its revocation by, or the competency of, the principal and note their findings in the medical record.

A health care surrogate designation must be reviewed to determine if it complies with statutory requirements relating to the execution and witnessing of a written document. The patient's capacity to make health care decisions should be evaluated and guidelines prescribed similar to those given in the hospital policy applying to the refusal of treatment by patients with and without decision-making capacity (**Form 1.3.1**). The policy also deals with the powers and restrictions relating to a surrogate or proxy's authority, a court review of his or her decisions, and revocation of his or her authority.

Among the procedures given are those for the assessment of the patient's capacity to make health care decisions and, if capacity is lacking, for the selection and notification of a surrogate or proxy. **Forms 1.3.2 and 1.3.3** provide such notifications. One of the potential proxies listed in some statutes, although last in the order of priority, is a close personal friend. The policy requires an affidavit to be signed by this individual setting forth that he or she is a friend of the patient, is familiar with the patient's beliefs and wishes, and is willing to be responsible for the patient's health care. **Form 3.3.2** offers such an affidavit.

3.4 STANDARDS FOR SURROGATE DECISION MAKING

As with the health care surrogate, the authority of a proxy begins when a patient is evaluated as lacking decision making capacity and continues until that capacity may be regained. Health care decisions by a proxy or surrogate may cover all matters relating to the health care of an incompetent patient. A refusal-of-treatment document to be signed by the proxy or surrogate is given in **Form 1.3.4**. It contains a release to the hospital and medical personnel from the results of refusing treatment. The document is to be signed by the attending physician and witnessed.

But before any health care decision can be made for an incompetent patient, one of two legal criteria set up by the courts for decision making by proxies or surrogates must be met. The first is the subjective test or "substituted judgment" criterion used by the *Quinlan* court and the majority of courts.[62] This criterion does not permit the surrogate decision maker to substitute his or her judgment for the patient's. The object is to determine the wants and needs of the patient and to decide on the course of action patients would have decided to take if they were competent. The decision maker stands in the shoes of the patient and must make the treatment decision the patient would have made even though the decision is different from what the decision maker would make and even if the decision seems wrong or foolish.

Most courts hold that in order for a substituted judgment to be made, it is imperative for the surrogate to know what a patient's personal decision would have been. In *Cruzan,* where Nancy Cruzan's parents were not allowed to make a treatment decision for her, substituted judgment was not possible because they could not meet Missouri's evidentiary standard and show by clear and convincing evidence what their daughter's decision would have been. Before incompetency, a patient may have expressed a personal decision to refuse life-sustaining treatment in several ways: a written or oral directive provided to a physician, family member, or friend might do so; the tenets of a patient's religion might imply it; or statements might have been made voicing the patient's views concerning medical treatment given to other patients, such as Paul Brophy's statements made to his wife when the *Quinlan* case was discussed. But while these may be evidence of the patient's wishes, their probative value will vary. A written advance directive—a living will, a durable power of attorney for health care, or a health care surrogate designation—would have the greatest value. If none has been made or one has been revoked, whatever the other evidence, written or oral, it should be reliable and strong enough to produce a firm conviction of what a patient would have decided before becoming incompetent.

The second standard is the objective test or "best interests" criterion, which is preferred by some courts over the subjective test when the evidence concerning a patient's intent to refuse or accept life-sustaining treatment is not strong or trustworthy enough for a surrogate to be sure of making the treatment decision a patient would have made. In this situation, life-sustaining treatment may be withdrawn or withheld from a patient if the benefits derived by the patient from continuing to live are clearly outweighed by the net burdens of life with treatment. The courts[63] using this test assume that patients would agree with treatment decisions that serve their best interests.

First in importance for surrogate decision making is promptness. The surrogate's decision about medical treatment for the incompetent should be made as expeditiously as possible, before a patient is forced to continue suffering as an object of unwanted medical technology and before a patient dies.

Second, the decision-making process should include all those individuals whose input and interests affect the decision—physicians, family, friends. But in the final analysis, the decision is made by the surrogate alone.

Third, in order to make a decision, the surrogate should obtain and consider all essential information, including the following: (1) whether there is a reasonable probability that the patient will recover competency and be able to exercise personally the right to accept or reject treatment; (2) whether the patient's physical condition is terminal; (3) where the subjective test for surrogate decision making is used, whether the evidence of what the patient would have wanted before becoming incompetent is sufficiently clear to enable the surrogate to make a substituted judgment; and (4) where the best-interests test is used, whether the burdens of treatment administered to the patient in terms of pain and suffering outweigh the benefits experienced by the patient.

To determine if a patient's physical condition is terminal or if he or she may recover capacity, the surrogate should have current medical input. Rather than oral information from physicians, the surrogate should ask for written medical evidence on which the surrogate can rely. Certificates or sworn statements from physicians should be secured. Such a document is provided in **Form 3.4.1**. It contains a documentation from a patient's attending physician and a consulting physician, such as a neurological specialist, certifying the existence of a terminal condition, which is defined in the language of an applicable state statute on advance directives either as a hopeless condition which, if not treated, will cause death or as a permanent vegetative state characterized by certain criteria. The certificate also describes what decision-making capacity consists of and whether or not the patient has it. For the best-interests test, a surrogate will also ask for medical evidence that treatment to the patient will not provide any net benefit but will only prolong the patient's pain and suffering, and for a determination of whether the pain can be reduced by drugs or other means short of stopping life-sustaining treatment.

4

Termination of Treatment

4.1 WITHHOLDING OR WITHDRAWING LIFE-SUSTAINING TREATMENT

When a patient does not have decision-making capacity, the attending physician and hospital staff should carry on extended consultations with the surrogate, proxy, family, and friends. At length, when a surrogate or proxy reasonably believes that he or she is making the same decision the patient would have made prior to the loss of decision-making capacity (if exercising substituted judgment), or that the degree of physical pain and suffering caused by further treatment and the degree of loss of dignity or humiliation caused by the treatment or condition might outweigh any physical pleasure, emotional enjoyment, or intellectual satisfaction life may offer the patient (if using the best-interests test), the surrogate or proxy may proceed to exercise the incompetent patient's right to forgo life-sustaining treatment. Courts have ruled that a surrogate's health care decisions include the refusal of life-sustaining treatment.[64] **Form 4.1.1** suggests a simple document to be signed by a surrogate designated by a patient that acknowledges consultation with the admitting physician and agreement with the withholding or withdrawing of life support. It is to be signed as well by the physician and by two individuals who have witnessed the consultation.

An alternate and more complete form, **Form 4.1.1.1**, provides a direction by a surrogate, court-appointed guardian, or proxy to withhold or withdraw life-sustaining treatment. It states that in the opinions of the attending and consulting physicians, the patient is terminally ill and is incapable of making health care decisions. The form can be modified if a statute permits this assessment by only the patient's attending physician. In the form the surrogate, guardian, or proxy directs the termination of life support according to the subjective judgment criterion and on the basis of his or her belief that the decision is the same the patient would have made had the patient been capable of deciding. The form is to be signed by the attending physician and two witnesses, and an interpreter if one was used. Where an advance directive has been made, the form is to be signed by the surrogate designated in a living will, health care surrogate designation, or durable power of attorney. Where no surrogate has been designated or no advance directive has been made by the patient, the form is to be signed by the guardian or proxy and the proxy's relationship to the patient is to be described.

4.2 HOSPITAL POLICIES AND PROCEDURES— WITHHOLDING OR WITHDRAWING LIFE-SUSTAINING TREATMENT FROM TERMINALLY ILL ADULT AND PEDIATRIC PATIENTS

Form 4.2.1 suggests a hospital procedure to be followed prior to making decisions about withholding or withdrawing life-sustaining procedures from terminally ill adult patients. The procedure deals with two classes of these patients: those with, and those without, advance directives.

For those who have executed advance directives, the instruments should be reviewed in accordance with the policy suggested by Form 3.3.1. Since under all living will laws a terminal condition, defined by the policy, must exist before life-sustaining treatment is withheld or withdrawn, the medical condition to which reference is made in a living will must be assessed. The procedure calls for separate examinations of the patient by the attending physician and a consulting physician and for the documentation of their findings in the patient's medical record. Each physician is to sign a certification in the form given in Form 3.4.1. A local statute may provide that their signed documentation constitutes a rebuttable presumption of the existence of the condition. A similar procedure is to be followed to determine whether a patient has recovered decision-making capacity. Separate evaluations of the patient by the attending physician and another physician are to be made and their agreement reached that decision-making capacity is absent. Their evaluations are to be entered in the medical record. As with a terminal condition, each physician completes a certification. If a health care surrogate has been designated in a living will or in another advance directive, written notice is to be given to that individual (Form 1.3.2). If no surrogate has been designated, a proxy will be selected and notified (Form 1.3.3) according to priorities listed in the hospital policy.

Noted above in connection with the refusal of medical treatment and an optional pregnancy clause (**Form 1.3.1.2**) was the principle enunciated by *Cruzan* and other cases that the right to refuse treatment was not destroyed by virtue of pregnancy. With respect to pregnant women who are terminally ill, three types of statutes adopt varying stances toward this principle and need to be consulted. The first type is represented by the living will statutes of ten states and the District of Columbia that are silent about pregnancy. The implication of this legislation is to grant pregnant women the right to refuse life-sustaining treatment in their advance directives. A hospital policy on withholding or withdrawing life-sustaining treatment, such as **Form 1.3.1**, the policy on refusal of treatment, and **Forms 1.1.4, 1.1.5,** and **1.2.1**, might simply not mention pregnancy and so permit pregnant women to forgo life support in their advance directives or through their surrogates or proxies. The second type of statute is illustrated by the living will laws of thirty-four states that do not permit a living will directing the withholding or withdrawing of life support to be carried out if the declarant is pregnant. Hospitals controlled by this legislation will reflect it in their policies. The third type of statutes on advance directives includes those that speak to the subject of pregnancy and allow a pregnant female to decide whether her surrogate will have authority to decline life support. If she has granted such authority to her surrogate (see **Form 2.3.7**), her advance directive will be honored. If she has made no advance directive, her proxy is not permitted to consent to the withholding or withdrawal of life support without court approval.

The policy described in **Form 4.2.1** (section I.B.3) follows this third type of legislation. If an advance directive has been made by a female of child-bearing age, the attending physician is to document in the medical record whether she is pregnant. The policy permits the pregnant patient's directions on forgoing life-sustaining treatment to be followed if the directive delegates authority to a surrogate to do so or if judicial approval has been received by a surrogate or proxy. If a pregnant female has not made an advance directive, her proxy cannot withhold or withdraw life-sustaining treatment in the absence of court approval. The life of the pregnant patient will be sustained until the fetus is viable. The policy (section II.B.3) directs the medical management of each case according to its merits and gives the attending physician access to the hospital's bioethics committee and legal counsel.

Generally, when a patient has no decision-making capacity, the physicians will consult at length with the surrogate, proxy, family, and friends. After such consultations, the surrogate or proxy may direct the withholding or withdrawal of life support by executing the documents suggested by **Forms 4.1.1** or **4.1.1.1**. The direction should be noted in the medical record. If no surrogate or proxy can be found, some statutes permit a hospital to proceed according to the directions given in the advance directive. The policy suggested provides for this eventuality.

The next-of-kin of a patient who has made an advance directive do not participate in end-of-life decisions. However, the policy provides also that attempts be made to keep them informed.

Once the decision has been made to terminate life-sustaining treatment, the attending physician is to write necessary orders to withhold or withdraw any treatment except palliative care. Whether and when a do-not-resuscitate or no-code-blue order is written are discussed in Section 5.1.

A common feature of living will statutes covers situations in which health providers are prevented by their values and beliefs from carrying out a patient's directions. The policy under consideration provides that if a patient is not an emergency case and has been notified of the hospital's policies about its beliefs, reasonable efforts will be made to transfer the patient to a provider who will honor them. The costs of the transfer will be paid by the provider. However, the patient's directions will be carried out by the provider if no transfer has been effected.

The procedure for patients who have no advance directive is the same with respect to evaluating the patient's physical condition and decision-making capacity. If a patient has such capacity, a request may be made for the patient to make an advance directive which will be supplied and made part of the medical record. If no advance directive is made or no health care surrogate designated, a proxy is to be selected from the priority list in the policy. If the patient is pregnant, the attending physician will have access to the hospital bioethics committee, an ad hoc committee, or hospital legal counsel. A decision of the proxy to terminate life support for a patient with no advance directive must meet either the substituted judgment or best-interests standard. In this policy, which follows the former, any decision by the proxy must be based on clear and convincing evidence that the decision is one which the patient would have made. If the decision is not, judicial review of the decision may be in order; otherwise, the proxy will complete **Form 4.1.1.1**. The provisions of the policy regarding the writing of physician's orders once the decision to terminate life support has been made are the same as in the case of a patient with an advance directive, as are the provisions regarding transfer of the patient if the provider cannot comply with the treatment decisions of the proxy or health care surrogate.

Form 4.2.2 provides a hospital policy for the termination of life-sustaining procedures for terminally ill pediatric patients.

Its procedures are the same as in the policy for adult patients, except for the following chief differences:

1. Since a minor does not have the capacity to make an advance directive, section I of the adult policy is omitted.

2. Section I.B.1 of the minor's policy differs from section II.B.1 of the adult's policy. The reference to recovering capacity is eliminated because the minor never had the capacity to make health care decisions. Section I.B.1 also requires documentation of the terminal condition on a different document, shown in **Form 4.2.3**, which eliminates the provisions regarding decision-making capacity to be found in the form certifying an adult patient's condition.

3. Section II.B.2 of the adult's policy is omitted for the same reason.

4. Section I.C.1 omits reference to an advance directive or health care surrogate and limits the appointment of a proxy to a guardian or a parent. (Provisions of sections II.D.b, c, e, f, g of the adult's policy are omitted.)

5. Section I.C.2 regarding documentation of the proxy's consent differs from sections II.D.2.a, b of the adult's policy because a minor lacks the capacity to make a decision, and in any event, it would be difficult to know the intentions and wishes of a child, in respect to terminating life-sustaining treatment. In the minor's policy, the proxy's consent following agreement with the attending physician requires that two witnesses be present at the consultation.

6. Section I.C.3, 4 refers to a request by a proxy to terminate life support, represented by **Form 4.2.4**. This differs from the form of request specified in sections II.D.3, 4 in that it omits reference to a lack of decision-making capacity since the minor never had such capacity.

7. In section I.D.2 the color of the no-code order becomes pink for the minor patient instead of blue as provided in section II.E.2 of the adult's policy.

8. Section I.E of the pediatric policy differs from section II.F of the adult's policy in that it omits references to a surrogate, to the receipt on admission of information relative to the hospital's policies, and to the wishes of the patient.

9. Section II.G of the adult's policy is omitted.

Physicians have reported a special emotion-laden problem in respect to the procedure given in sections I.C.2, 3, 4, dealing with documenting and signing the proxy's consent. Even after extended and careful discussions with parents

of terminally ill children and the parents' intellectual acceptance of and oral
consent to the termination of life-sustaining treatment for a child, in their
overwhelming grief or guilt, they are reluctant to or cannot sign **Form 4.2.4**
to request termination of the treatment. For them, the document represents
the child's death warrant. Yet without their voluntary written consent,
physicians are fearful of proceeding with termination at the same time they
believe that they cannot continue treatment which is futile. In the light of
this problem, a hospital may wish to adopt a policy which will allow the
doctrine of informed consent to be respected and futile procedures to be
ceased while medical personnel are still protected. An alternative clause which
permits the attending physician to document the situation in the progress
notes is provided in **Form 4.2.3.1** to replace the one in section I.C.3.

To the already difficult situations involving the termination of life-sustaining treatment, another may be added—one involving older minors. All
statutes authorizing advance directives limit the right to make them to
competent adults. Unemancipated individuals below the age of majority are
not considered competent by the law to give informed consent to or to refuse
medical or surgical treatment, including the stoppage of life-sustaining
treatment. The consent of a proxy or parent is always required, as it is in the
policy proposed in **Form 4.2.2**. The requirement is consonant with the law
relating to all individuals below the age of eighteen in most states (twenty-one
in others). However, while few people question the wisdom and operation of
the law's presumption that infants and very young children lack the competence to give informed consent or refusal to medical treatment, the presumption weakens with teenagers. The law does not apply to those who are
emancipated. However, a recent Florida case involving a mature teenager who
lived at home and was not emancipated has further weakened the law's
presumption.

In June 1984, fifteen-year-old Benny Arigo refused to take a medication
which might have prevented his body from rejecting a transplanted liver
because the drug caused him pain and intense headaches. Workers from the
Department of Health and Rehabilitative Services, denying that he had any
right to refuse the medication, forcibly removed the screaming, struggling
boy from his home, strapped him to a stretcher, and took him to Jackson
Memorial Hospital in Miami where the prescribed medicine was to be
administered. However, after a judge questioned Benny and found him to be
capable of understanding his condition, his right to refuse life-sustaining
treatment was upheld and he was released from the hospital. Before he died
in August 1994, Benny appeared on ABC's "Prime Time Live" as a symbol
to others of someone who calmly made a choice to live, and die, in his own
way ("Teen Shunned Medication," 1994).

This and similar precedents may suggest that when physicians encounter unemancipated teenage minors who, as Benny Arigo did, appear mature, able to understand an explanation of their physical conditions and the proposed procedures, and capable of making health care decisions—even those reaching as far as the termination of life support—a hospital may wish to consult with legal counsel about the legal necessity of a proxy's consent. They may also wish to consider adopting a policy that either: (1) recognizes the desirability of allowing a mature minor to participate in a decision concerning the withholding or withdrawal of life-sustaining treatment, although the ultimate legal consent will continue to rest with the proxy, or (2) dispenses with the selection and consent of a proxy and accepts the consent of such a minor as sufficient and valid. An optional clause is provided for the former in **Form 4.2.3.2** which might be inserted as a new section I.D in **Form 4.2.2**. The present sections D, E, F, and G would be relettered E, F, G, and H, respectively. An optional clause for the latter found in **Form 4.2.3.3** might be inserted as a new section I.C.1 in place of the existing sections I.C.1, 2, 3, 4 so that all references to a proxy are eliminated. The new section would be entitled "Minor's Decision to Withdraw or Withhold Life-Sustaining Treatment."

5

Withholding
Cardiopulmonary Resuscitation

5.1 DO-NOT-RESUSCITATE ORDER

"Code blue" (for adults) and "code pink" (for infants) signify that cardiopulmonary resuscitation (CPR) measures are to be administered if a healthy patient suffers cardiac or respiratory arrest in order to prevent sudden and unexpected death, to restore cardiac function or to support ventilation, and to revive the patient. Because patients do not have the ability to make known their wishes concerning CPR when such arrest occurs, their consent to these measures is implied since the situation constitutes an emergency. The measures are routinely followed in a health care facility and are to be distinguished from other measures because no physician's order is needed to administer them. They are terminated or withheld, however, if a "no code" order has been written or a do-not-resuscitate (DNR) order is prepared by the attending physician stating that in the event of cardiac or respiratory arrest, cardiopulmonary resuscitation is to be withheld.

Because the issuance of the DNR order continues to cause some of the greatest ethical concerns in the practice of medicine, animated discussions took place at our hospital's ethics committee which revolved around the issue of futility. Several physicians stated that when they believed that cardiopulmonary resuscitation would be futile and could not benefit the patient, they made unilateral decisions to withhold CPR, wrote do-not-resuscitate orders without offering resuscitation as an option to, or obtaining the consent of, the patient, surrogate, or proxy; documented the reasons for the order in the medical record; and then informed patients, surrogates, or proxies of their decisions.

The views and procedures expressed by these doctors are supported by considerable legal and medical authority. In *In re Dinnerstein*,[65] where a sixty-seven-year-old comatose woman had Alzheimer's disease and was being sustained by a nasogastric tube, the family and attending physician wanted a DNR order but were concerned about its legality. The Massachusetts Appeals Court, saying that the order did not involve life-sustaining treatment, upheld the issuance of the order as peculiarly within the competence of the medical profession and attending physician, not the court, although it was subject to court review if the physician failed to exercise the degree of care and skill of the average qualified practitioner.

Support also comes from a long-standing ethical principle that futile intervention is never obligatory for the physician. Most physicians, an opinion of the Council on Ethical and Judicial Affairs of the American Medical Association (1991), and some commentators (Blackhall, 1987) agree that it is within the right of physicians to determine, as they would determine any other medical procedure, if CPR is medically appropriate. On the ground of futility, they do not require a physician to offer a procedure to a patient, or obtain a patient's consent for it or for a DNR order, or administer any intervention in spite of a patient's request personally or in an advance directive, if the intervention is judged by the physician to be futile.

The word *futility* is in constant use in medical circles but there is little attempt to clarify it and limit it to clearly defined medical situations. If, for example, the physician's judgment not to administer treatment or offer patient, surrogate, or proxy the choice of treatment were limited to cases in which no physiologic benefit can reasonably be expected, its meaning seems clear. For example, the goal of CPR is to restore cardiac and respiratory function and if a return of functioning cannot be expected on rational grounds and medical evidence, then CPR may be said to be physiologically futile. An intervention may also be clearly futile when it has already failed in a patient or has no pathophysiologic rationale. Otherwise, to what does futility relate, in whose judgment and by whose values? It becomes an abstract notion, one which physicians themselves conceive differently and on which they cannot always agree. Between patient and physician, there may be similar disagreement. From the medical point of view, CPR is considered futile if a patient's life will only be prolonged briefly after cardiac arrest. A short period of survival is not enough to warrant its use (Bedell, Delbanco, et al., 1983). But from the patient's perspective, if CPR will allow him or her to continue to live for another hour, day, month, or year, it may not be futile (Youngner, 1988) because it may give God time to work a miracle. In one case a woman insisted on CPR because she had seen with her own eyes how her mother with an inoperable brain tumor had been the beneficiary of a miraculous cure deemed impossible by the mother's doctors. For other dying patients, CPR is not futile if it allows their coping mechanism to help them delay and deny the reality of death. Many observers, therefore, reject futility as a meaningless, value-laden concept which is not objective (Truog et al., 1992).

If a unilateral decision to stop or withhold CPR were to be acceptable and legitimate, it would only be in the strict and objective sense of physiological futility, which relates to the reasonable probability that a treatment will accomplish a specific physiologic objective and benefit (Lo, 1991). But whether futility is used in this strict sense or in looser and less objective ways in order to allow unilateral decisions by physicians to enter DNR orders in the medical record or override requests for interventions made by patients, surrogates, or proxies, it appears to be a throwback to the paternalistic era of "doctor knows best." It becomes a serious question whether what is done in the name of futility is consistent with the principles of self-determination, privacy, and liberty interest which courts have consistently upheld since the 1970s and which permit competent adults, according to their own values and preferences, or their surrogates or proxies, to decide whether to have medical procedures provided, withheld, or withdrawn.

There is a clear conflict here, and courts are the places in which conflicts are resolved. It is a curious fact, however, that U.S. courts have never directly adjudicated the question of hospitals and physicians refusing on the ground of futility to provide treatment for a patient in the face of demands by the patient or family that it be provided. They were, therefore, special legal events when two cases were brought to courts by hospitals and physicians who petitioned for decisions that would relieve them of furnishing medical treatment requested on behalf of patients and which the hospitals and physicians judged to be ethically or medically inappropriate.

In 1991, the question arose in the Minnesota case of Helen Wanglie, an elderly woman in a persistent vegetative state, who was hospitalized in Hennepin County Medical Center. The case was the opposite of the *Quinlan* and *Cruzan*-type cases, in which surrogates and proxies fought to have treatment of incompetent patients discontinued or withheld. Oliver Wanglie, the patient's husband and surrogate, fought to have the hospital continue mechanical ventilation and intensive care for his wife. The hospital, however, claiming that such continued treatment was inappropriate and futile, petitioned a court for the appointment of a conservator because Wanglie was not acting in his wife's best interest. Although some observers disagreed (Callahan, 1991), the medical world applauded the hospital's action in bringing the matter to court (Rie, 1991). But the court did not rule on this aspect of the Wanglie case. It ruled only that the evidence did not show that Oliver Wanglie was not capable of discharging his duties as his wife's surrogate; the hospital's petition was therefore denied, and Wanglie remained his wife's representative.[66]

In the second case, an anencephalic baby, known as Baby "K," was born at Fairfax Hospital in Falls Church, Virginia, in 1992. Anencephaly is a condition in which the major part of the brain, skull case, and scalp are missing. Only the brain stem and spinal cord are present. Anencephalic infants can have brain stem or spinal reflexes for some days or weeks but 95 percent of those who are live-born die within a week of birth. Baby "K" had difficulty in breathing and had been given mechanical ventilation. When the physicians wanted to discontinue the ventilation, the mother objected and would not allow them to do so. The hospital, maintaining that it and the physicians were not obligated to prescribe or render medical treatment that was medically or ethically inappropriate, petitioned a federal court for a declaration to this effect. After the trial court ruled against the hospital, the hospital appealed to the Fourth Circuit court. The appellate court, by a two-to-one opinion,[67] affirmed the lower court only on the grounds that the Emergency Medical Treatment and Woman in Active Labor Act of 1986 required the hospital and physicians to provide the ventilatory treatment requested by the mother because the child's respiratory problems constituted an emergency condition. The case was decided on the basis of the statute.

In both cases, the medical coummunity had hoped that at last a court would rule that the medical profession is under no obligation to provide health care that is morally repugnant to physicians and is medically inappropriate. But the futility question, which had poked its head up shyly in both cases, disappeared from view and was not decided again.

The debate over the principle of autonomy can be placed on two levels, philosophical and political (Callahan, 1991). On the philosophical level, it may be possible to determine that, on scientific grounds, a particular treatment for a particular patient will be useless. On the political level, the dispute is whether physicians may make unilateral decisions about treatment considered futile or whether patients or families make the final decision. Callahan refers to this as "the historical struggle about expertise and democracy" (Callahan, 1991:91). Several fingers point to an end of the struggle and a victory by the medical profession. The unilateral issuance by physicians of a DNR order without presenting it as an option to a patient has been and continues to be a frequent and routine occurrence (Lipton, 1986). The validity of unilateral medical decision making based on the futility principle still has not been raised in and addressed by the courts in a malpractice suit or invoked in a criminal charge. The "doctor knows best" practice is not only strongly endorsed by the AMA and many in the medical profession; it is also supported by legislators. In one state, for example, an advance directive statute was enacted in 1992 that defined an advance directive as including a do-not-resuscitate order[68] and that further defined a do-not-resuscitate order as one that documented instructions by a patient.[69] To unilaterally issue a do-not-resuscitate order without a patient's instructions was to flirt with malpractice or criminal liability. Democracy appeared the victor in the struggle with expertise; patient autonomy seemed to be affirmed. But in 1994, the legislature, apparently convinced that physicians should not be forced to provide care judged futile by them, deleted these definitions.

Even if it is accepted that "doctor knows best" with respect to the DNR order, physicians nevertheless ought to hold discussions with their patients about CPR and the DNR order. Yet studies suggest that few physicians are disposed to talking with patients about the DNR order (Bedell and Delbanco, 1984). However, now that the Patient Self-Determination Act (see Section 6.1) requires health care facilities to apprise patients of their rights under the laws of their states to refuse or accept life-sustaining treatment and make advance directives, physicians may be more disposed to starting discussions regarding CPR with patients being admitted for surgical care or medical treatment. To further these discussions and to help hospitals supply information to patients as the act mandates, **Form 5.1.1** provides a question and answer format to advise patients about CPR and the DNR order.

Discussions with patients should be held routinely and initiated early on when patients are lucid. In their discussions, physicians should try to elicit from patients their wishes with respect to CPR, especially in the cases of hospitalized chronically ill, terminally ill, and elderly patients who probably will suffer respiratory failure or cardiac arrest (Ruark et al., 1988). The physician should ascertain beforehand whether the application of CPR is medically appropriate for a patient. Should the determination be that CPR would be beneficial, the patient may nevertheless choose to decline it, whether because of a chronic medical condition or for some other reason. For this purpose, a patient may sign **Form 5.1.2**, which is a specific refusal of resuscitation and which releases the hospital from liability. Alternatively, the patient with decision-making capacity might sign a general refusal-of-treatment form (**Form 1.2.1**). A patient's surrogate or proxy would sign the general refusal-of-treatment provided by **Form 1.3.4**.

If the physician determines that the application of CPR is medically inappropriate, clearly futile, and harmful to the patient, the physician should be candid and detailed in explaining the rationale for no resuscitation to the patient, surrogate, or proxy, including the seriousness of the patient's medical condition and the risks. To allow an informed decision to be made, the physician should also explain the significant finding that CPR has a poor success ratio for adult patients—only about 15 percent of these in hospitals who receive CPR survive (Bedell, Delbanco, et al., 1983) and none survive who have metastatic cancer (Faber-Langendoen, 1991). Even if resuscitation restores basic functions, patients should know that it still may result in severe damage to the brain or other organs and that it will lead them to an intensive care unit or cardiac care unit where, even in the most humane unit, the invasiveness of treatment, constant noise, and limits on visits by the family can be nightmarish (Ruark et al., 1988).

During the discussions, physicians should also make it clear that if a DNR order is issued, other vigorous support will continue. This is important not only for patients; it is a matter that ought to be understood by medical professionals as well. As the meaning of futility is not clear, so the meaning of a DNR order is not clear to many medical personnel. Although the DNR order relates only to the stoppage in initiating or carrying out cardiopulmonary measures for patients who have suffered cardiac or pulmonary arrest, it is often misunderstood by health professionals as a mandate to restrict or preclude procedures and to do nothing. Even if a patient consents to a DNR order, its issuance does not limit or eliminate support in other therapeutic care. Patients will still receive dialysis, pain control, supportive comfort and care, intensive care, transfusions, antibiotics, and other therapeutic interventions.

If a patient is suffering from a terminal illness, lacks decision-making capacity, and has rejected CPR in a living will, that document will give the patient DNR status. In the absence of a terminal condition, a patient without decision-making capacity but with a living will that rejects CPR is not in DNR status. A patient with decision-making capacity, however, can agree that there is to be no resuscitation. Oral agreement can be given in the presence of two adult witnesses. In lieu of **Form 5.1.2**, a written consent to no resuscitation to be signed by the patient is suggested in **Form 5.1.3**. This same form, instead of **Form 1.3.4**, can also be signed by the surrogate or proxy if the patient has no decision-making capacity or if a physician determines that the well-being of the patient would be adversely affected by a discussion of the patient's medical condition and CPR. While a DNR order issued by a physician and entered in the medical record may stipulate merely that no CPR is to be given, **Form 5.1.4** contains a more detailed type of order which deals with specific procedures to be withheld.

5.2 HOSPITAL POLICY AND PROCEDURES—DO-NOT-RESUSCITATE ORDER

Hospitals are obligated to have written policies on the DNR order in order to be accredited by the Joint Commission on Accreditation of Healthcare Organizations (1987). The Council on Ethical and Judicial Affairs of the AMA (1991) also encourages revision of DNR policies and physician education about the part they play in the decision-making process.

The DNR order occupies a war zone in medical practice. Although the AMA and several authorities are opposed to permitting patients to be involved in decisions whether or not to issue it, the attitudes of many physicians are in conflict over the issue. Illustrative of the conflict is the split vote cast by the nineteen members of our ethics committee when the time came to adopt a DNR policy: ten voted for one kind and nine for another. Since physician opinion is sharply divided, two alternative forms of policies are supplied which give hospitals a choice and which may provide some guidance for the development or revision of their policies.

The policy offered by **Form 5.2.1** is highly sensitive to the principles of autonomy and informed consent, to possible malpractice or criminal liability, and to current medical ethics (American College of Physicians, 1989). It recognizes that the DNR order rests on the consent of the patient and that the physician is not the sole decision maker.

It assumes that CPR will be initiated in every case of cardiac or pulmonary arrest except when DNR or no-code orders have been issued. After providing definitions of CPR and the DNR order, it calls for the attending physician to determine the medical appropriateness of CPR and to hold candid discussions with patients concerning CPR that are sufficient to permit informed consent. As a safeguard, a registered nurse or two witnesses are to be present during these discussions.

The physician may not issue the DNR order unilaterally. The concurrence of the patient, surrogate, or proxy with the withholding of CPR is required. A living will which has rejected CPR provides a DNR status to a terminally ill patient who lacks decision-making capacity. If the declaration does not do so and a patient with decision-making capacity decides to forgo CPR, the living will can and should be amended. A patient who is not terminally ill and has decision-making capacity may refuse CPR. The refusal may be given by the patient orally before two adult witnesses, one of whom is the physician, or it may be given in a written statement (**Form 5.1.2**) signed by the patient in the presence of two adult witnesses and signed also by the attending physician. An interpreter is also to sign when a patient is not English-speaking. Patients may also use **Form 1.2.1** to reject resuscitation.

Should an attending physician evaluate a patient as obviously incapable of making informed decisions, or if capacity is questionable and the attending physician and another physician agree that a patient lacks decision-making capacity or will be adversely affected by a discussion of CPR, the patient's representatives may refuse CPR. **Form 1.3.4** may be signed by a surrogate or proxy after full explanation by the physician. The form is to be completed also by two witnesses, the attending physician and an interpreter, if necessary. In case a physician believes that a refusal of CPR by a patient, surrogate, or proxy is medically inappropriate, machinery is described for further investigation of the rationale behind the refusal and consultations with facilitators. If no resolution of the disagreement is forthcoming, the physician's right to withdraw from the case is recognized.

In cases of adult patients, a hospital may encounter an emotion-laden situation similar to that when parents cannot sign a form to terminate life-sustaining treatment for a child. The representatives of an adult patient for whom a DNR order is to be issued may not be able to bring themselves to sign a refusal of resuscitative treatment although they are in agreement with the attending physician that application of CPR is inappropriate. The hospital may therefore wish to adopt a policy similar to the one dealing with the documentation of the proxy's or surrogate's consent when life-sustaining treatment for pediatric patients is to be withdrawn or withheld. **Form 5.2.1.1** provides an optional clause to follow the clause in section 9, under which the attending physician may document the situation and the oral consent of the patient's representatives.

Form 5.2.1.2 provides a guide to progress notes to be made by a physician relating to discussions with the patient, surrogate, or proxy and information about the patient's decision-making capacity, if in doubt, and about any adverse effects from a disclosure of the patient's medical status. A registered nurse should also sign the progress notes as witness to the discussion if **Form 5.1.2** consenting to the withholding of CPR is not signed by the patient and nurse.

The DNR order must be reduced to a formal written order whose meaning is brought home to the hospital staff. Reducing it to writing puts the staff on notice that they are not to attempt to revive the patient, and when they follow it, it also protects them from malpractice claims that they did not do their duty to revive the patient. The DNR order, however, does not obviate the need for other therapeutic or supportive care.

In case a patient refuses to concur with the physician's judgment and to consent to a DNR order when the physician believes that CPR is futile, the policy does not permit patients to impose their values on the physician. The physician cannot be ethically obligated and should not be coerced to administer a procedure which violates his or her morals. The moral obligation of the physician is recognized by the policy. It recommends an explanation to the patient of the physician's medical opinion and consultations with facilitators because frequently they result in agreement by patients or their representatives to the DNR order. If these alternatives do not resolve matters, provision is made for the physician's withdrawal from the case and transfer of the patient to another physician (President's Commission, 1983).

Provisions also appear in the policy to deal with the revocation of a DNR order by the patient, surrogate, or proxy if situations arise that may make revocation of the DNR order appropriate, such as an improvement in the patient's condition, the discovery of an error in the original medical diagnosis, or the development of a new therapy for the patient's condition. The policy describes the steps to be taken in the event of revocation and of withdrawal by the physician who judges CPR futile if consultations are not successful. The policy also provides that situations may arise when the physician will recommend revocation of the DNR order. But if no agreement can be reached with the patient, proxy, or surrogate regarding the recommended revocation, provision is made for consultation and, if that fails, for withdrawal by the physician.

The policy recognizes the possibility that after a DNR order has been issued, situations may arise which make it appropriate to suspend the order. An example is a medical problem that can be corrected easily, such as a transurethral prostatic resection in a patient with cancer. The policy does not accept limited, slow, and chemical codes (i.e., cursory procedures that fail to attain full CPR) as proper medical practice and goes on to provide for DNR orders which are temporarily suspended.

A hospital may wish to consider adding an optional clause, suggested by **Form 5.2.1.3**, to this policy in order to expedite guardianship proceedings for patients who lack decision-making capacity, who have made no advance directives, and for whom no person can be found to act as proxy. A legal guardian will be able to consent to a DNR order.

An alternate and much briefer policy is suggested by **Form 5.2.2**. It takes the approach that the decision to withhold or stop CPR procedures is strictly a medical judgment and that patients are not to participate in decisions concerning the DNR order. It is a highly practical policy in two respects. First, it is in accord with what is actually going on in hospitals. Studies suggest that 75 percent of deaths in hospitals are preceded by DNR orders but that no more than 22 percent of the patients dying participate in the decisions to issue them (Bedell, Pelle, et al., 1986). Second, although thousands of malpractice suits and many cases involving life-sustaining treatment have passed through the legal system, there has been an apparent failure or reluctance in the courts thus far to deal with the question of unilateral DNR orders based on futility. The policy is therefore willing to roll the dice and bet with some assurance of winning either that there will be no lawsuit for malpractice or criminal prosecution brought against the hospital or its personnel, or that if court proceedings are begun, the issue of futility will continue to be bypassed by judges in favor of other reasons for their rulings.

Like the policy in **Form 5.2.1**, this one calls for CPR by the staff when a patient suffers a cardiac or respiratory arrest and provides that these procedures will be stopped or withheld when the attending physician has entered a DNR order. But unlike the other policy, **Form 5.2.2** is based on the principle that physicians are not morally obligated to provide a treatment that is futile. The policy, however, attempts to clarify the meaning of futility by providing illustrations of it for the guidance of physicians. It requires them to detail in the progress notes the medical basis for the patient's DNR status and to explain it to the patient, surrogate, or proxy. When an intervention is futile, the physician may issue the DNR order without offering the choice of CPR to the patient, surrogate, or proxy and without getting his or her permission. The physician need only consult with the primary service—the caregivers to whom the patient went initially for medical care. A DNR order may also be entered on the request of a patient, surrogate, or proxy, although the request is made subject to consultation procedures to be sure that it is an appropriate request.

The alternate policy requires that a written DNR order be issued by the attending physician and entered in the patient's medical record. But consider this case: It is 3 o'clock in the morning. The attending physician, at home in bed, answers a telephone call from the hospital. His patient's heart has stopped. No written DNR order has been issued previously and placed in the patient's chart. May the physician give a DNR order over the telephone? In recognition of these circumstances, the hospital may want to consider a carefully limited exception to its procedural requirement. The exception should be permitted only if certain stipulated criteria are met. One such criterion might be that an outpatient prehospital do-not-resuscitate order (see Section 5.3) had been executed by the physician and patient before the patient's admission or readmission to the hospital. Another criterion justifying the exception might be that in the months prior to the patient's admission to the hospital, the patient had been under the care of the physician who had determined that CPR would be futile and had provided the patient, surrogate, or proxy with an explanation of the medical basis for futility. The exception should oblige the physician to document in the progress notes, within twenty-four hours after the oral DNR order, the reasons for it and whether it has met one of the prescribed criteria. The documentation should be made whether or not the patient has died. If adopted, the exception should be inserted in the alternate policy as a new paragraph 4d.

5.3 PREHOSPITAL DO-NOT-RESUSCITATE ORDER

A patient is terminally ill. Her physicians decide that nothing more can be done for her medically. She knows that she is dying and asks to be sent home where she can die in the company of her family. She had prepared a living will because she wanted her family and physicians to know that she wanted to die naturally, and among the forms of life support she specifically refused was CPR. She was at home for two weeks when she suffered cardiac arrest. A friend visiting her became frantic and called 911. Within minutes emergency medical services personnel were on the scene. They found that the woman's heart had stopped and began to administer CPR. The friend shouted to them to stop. She showed them the woman's living will. But they refused. Were they right? Did they violate the patient's wishes?

They had no choice. The goal of the emergency medical services (EMS) program is to provide basic and advanced life support to try to restore breathing and circulation. EMS personnel are obligated to administer CPR in every instance and to refuse to honor even a living will specifically rejecting CPR that was executed by the person whose life they are attempting to save. A living will is effective only if a patient is in a terminal condition. EMS personnel cannot make this diagnosis.

But many people, among them the elderly, desire only to be left alone to die in peace at home without being forced into receiving unwanted resuscitative measures instituted by EMS personnel. Therefore, the statutes of some states were amended with provisions for prehospital do-not-resuscitate orders to allow EMS personnel, although obliged to save and maintain life, to respect the wishes of those who choose to expire in their homes. The statutes do not grant EMS personnel authority to honor living wills; they allow them to honor a prehospital do-not-resuscitate order which constitutes a determination regarding the patient's physical condition and course of treatment. The order, which must be signed by the attending physician, directs EMS personnel to withhold CPR although they may provide the patient with limited medical care when they respond to a call for assistance. The physician must state in the order that he or she has documented in the patient's medical record whether or not the patient has decision-making capacity. If the patient is capable of providing informed consent, the patient must also sign the order directing that CPR not be administered and his or her signature must be witnessed. If the patient lacks decision-making capacity, the physician must indicate in the order whether an advance directive has been completed that forgoes life-sustaining treatment. If one has been completed, the document must be attached to the order and the appointed surrogate must sign the order directing that CPR not be administered to the patient. Should no advance directive have been completed by the patient, a judicially appointed guardian or proxy must sign the order to direct EMS personnel not to initiate CPR. The order must be presented to EMS personnel when they respond to a call. A prehospital DNR order is offered by **Form 5.3.1**. As an alternative to the prehospital order, a patient may wear an official DNR identification bracelet, which is as valid as the prehospital order itself and which has to be honored by EMS personnel if presented to them.

6

Autonomy and
the Federal Government

6.1 PATIENT SELF-DETERMINATION ACT

The functions of courts are judicial and not political, but their decisions frequently bring about political repercussions and alterations of public policy. Some of these had a distinct negative effect when state laws or acts of Congress of great social or economic importance were invalidated. The Dred Scott decision,[70] which held the Missouri Compromise invalid, helped bring on the Civil War, and the invalidation of the National Recovery Act,[71] which Congress had passed to bring the country out of the Great Depression, severely hurt government plans and policy. On the other hand, recent decisions in the medical field have been positive in character. In some the courts encouraged the passage of beneficial new laws to guide patients and courts in regard to life-sustaining treatment.[72] Others, such as *Quinlan*, produced living will statutes on the state level, while on the federal level, *Cruzan* influenced Congress to enact the Patient Self-Determination Act (PSDA), also known as the Omnibus Budget Reconciliation Act of 1990.[73] The act was the first legislation to make the federal government a powerful force in the campaign to educate the public about patient autonomy and the advance directives they can make—living wills, health care surrogate designations, and durable powers of attorney for health care—to ensure that their autonomy will continue to be respected even when they have lost decision-making capacity. As its title suggests, the aim of the act is to bring home to every individual the basic Anglo-American concept of self-determination and his or her right to refuse life-sustaining treatment and to make advance directives. It was not intended to create any new rights but merely to educate patients about their existing rights. Nor was the object to force patients to make advance directives; rather, it was only to motivate them to do so.

Congress required the U.S. Department of Health and Human Services to promote a national program to apprise the general public and recipients of Social Security benefits of their twin rights regarding treatment and advance directives. It imposed other requirements on all health care facilities in receipt of Medicare or Medicaid funds, including hospitals, nursing homes, hospices, home health agencies, and prepaid health maintenance organizations. One requirement is to provide all patients with written information explaining their rights under the statutory or case law of their state to accept or refuse medical or surgical treatment, the sorts of advance directives they could make, and the written policies maintained to implement patients' rights. Such information is to be provided by hospitals when patients are admitted, when patients are enrolled by prepaid health maintenance organizations, when patients first receive care from hospices, and before they receive care from a home health agency or nursing home. In addition, the PSDA requires provider organizations to document in the patient's medical records whether or not an advance directive has been executed and to maintain written policies and procedures to implement patients' rights to accept or refuse treatment and to make advance directives. Continued participation in the federal Medicare and Medicaid programs is conditioned upon fulfilling the PSDA's requirements.

The practice of hospitals with respect to when and how to comply with PSDA seems to vary. In addition to providing the information at the time of admission, a few may also supply it to patients by playing audio tapes in waiting rooms, by sending it via its closed-circuit television network to their rooms, or by placing written material in the rooms. Basically, the information consists of a description in writing of the law of the state regarding the rights of patients to make health care decisions and advance directives and regarding the policy of the health care facility about advance directives. It should be couched in language readily understandable by the public. Different examples of these descriptions in the form of a single sheet or a brochure are offered here to guide a hospital as it ascertains the laws of its state and prepares its own form that conforms to these laws. Form 6.1.1 is an example of a statement on a single sheet of paper that might be provided to patients concerning their rights to accept or refuse treatment and to formulate advance directives. Form 6.1.2 is one example of a brochure that might be furnished to patients to explain why advance directives were invented and the three forms they take.

The PSDA does not apply to individual practitioners. Although physicians are not legally obliged to do so, they might consider supplying information to their patients to make them aware of their rights regarding medical treatment and advance directives. Brief statements posted or made available in leaflets or pamphlets in their offices are suggested in **Form 6.1.3**, which provides optional clauses depending on whether physicians are or are not willing to honor advance directives to terminate life-sustaining treatment.

When it was enacted, the act was criticized on many grounds (Berger, 1993:124–126), the question of timing being one of them. Introducing patients to their rights when they are admitted to a hospital could not have been timed or conceived more badly. Admission is not the time to try to educate people who are sick, frightened, or under stress. One more document among the rain of other papers that descends on patients through admissions virtually guarantees that it will be ignored. The notion of having an unskilled and uncaring employee in the admissions office discuss advance directives with patients and their options regarding medical treatment also seems to guarantee that the act will fail; it makes discussion of these matters an institutional and bureaucratic one instead of a professional one. Patients need to give thought to, and make decisions about, treatment and advance directives prior to their admission into a hospital and before a critical illness, and their physicians, not admissions clerks, should help them.

During the three years since the federal law became effective, it has become clear that criticisms of it were justified. It has had little effect in increasing public awareness or promoting the use of advance directives. For example, after the hospital ethics committee on which I serve requested the quality manager of our hospital to monitor the effectiveness of its policies and procedures in compliance with the act, she had patients interviewed. The findings revealed that fewer than 1 percent of patients understood or were aware of the advance directives booklets or information sheets provided to them at the time of admission.

Two steps might be taken by health care institutions to increase the effectiveness of the act. One is to initiate follow-up procedures in which patients' representatives, social workers, trained volunteers, or members of hospital ethics committees visit patients after they have reached their units. The purposes of this step are to: (1) determine if patients received the written information mandated by the PSDA; (2) determine whether patients made an advance directive previously, wished to change it, or gave a copy of it to admissions; (3) give patients who had not made any advance directive the opportunity to ask questions; (4) provide patients with copies of advance directives to execute if they desire to do so and to obtain completed copies; and (5) allow patients to designate health care surrogates. **Form 6.1.4** provides a checklist for the hospital representative to follow, complete, sign, and place in the patient's chart.

It is apparent that the time to educate people about their rights to a voice in their medical treatment and to make advance directives is before they come to a health care facility. A community outreach program, consisting of trained speakers conducting free face-to-face discussions in the communities served by health care providers, would be more effective than handing out forms to patients on admission. These discussions would help people think about the issues, encourage them to initiate discussions with their physicians, and help them to understand how to complete advance directives which allow them to take control of their own care and participate in medical decision making. The program would not only carry out the basic thrust of the PSDA, which is to educate the public, it would conform to another of its requirements which many institutions seem to have ignored: "to provide [individually or with others] for education for . . . the community on issues concerning advance directives."[74]

6.2 HOSPITAL POLICY AND PROCEDURES—PATIENT SELF-DETERMINATION ACT

To comply with the PSDA requirement of a policy implementing advance directives and the acceptance or refusal of treatment, hospitals wishing to adopt a written policy and procedures which spell out the institution's policy might wish to consider **Form 6.2.1**, which is an attempt at compliance with the act.

The policy provided incorporates some relevant hospital policies previously mentioned which recognize the rights to refuse medical treatment by a patient with decision-making capacity or by a surrogate or proxy when such capacity is lacking (**Form 1.3.1**) and the right of a competent adult to make an advance directive (**Form 3.3.1**). The policy also sets up procedures for providing information to in-patients upon admission. If it is ascertained that an advance directive has been made, the procedures previously authorized by a prior policy (**Form 3.3.1**) are followed for its documentation, and procedures authorized by another policy (**Form 4.2.1**) are followed for terminating life-sustaining procedures. If no advance directive has been made, patients will be supplied with more information and encouraged to learn about them. In the absence of a directive, the termination of life-sustaining treatment will be governed by the procedures described in **Form 4.2.1**. The policy also contains provisions relating to the transfer of patients, the immunity from liability of health providers who comply with an advance directive, and the availability to patients of hospital policies dealing with the implementation of the rights of patients.

II

**MEDICOLEGAL FORMS
AND HOSPITAL POLICIES**

FORM 1.1.1
HOSPITAL POLICY AND PROCEDURES—
OBTAINING INFORMED CONSENT

POLICY

Health care is predicated on informed consent obtained by a medical professional prior to initiating any procedures from a patient or, if a patient lacks decision-making capacity, from a legitimate proxy. Such consent is to be obtained only after the patient has been fully informed and understands (1) his or her diagnosis; (2) the nature of the proposed treatment or procedure; (3) its benefits and risks; (4) alternative therapies and their benefits and risks; and (5) what may happen during the recuperation process after the procedure or treatment and what may happen if the proposed course of action is not followed. In an emergency life-threatening situation, however, where there is substantial evidence of the impairment of the patient's decision-making capacity, the physician may implement treatment without the prior consent of the patient. *Physician* means the admitting, attending, or treating physician.

Informed consent will be obtained in accordance with the following procedure.

PROCEDURE

Whenever the term *patient* is used, it is intended, if the patient is impaired or lacking in decision-making capacity, to include the patient's health care surrogate (if the patient has designated such a person to make health care decisions) or a legitimate proxy (if the patient has not designated a surrogate or the surrogate is not willing or able to perform his or her duties).

1. An informed consent form must be signed for all invasive diagnostic procedures or surgical procedures.

   A form documenting that the patient has given a valid informed consent must be signed by the patient and must be signed by a witness. This form must then be placed in the patient's chart.

   A patient's mark (x) must be witnessed by two registered nurses.

   Telephoned informed consents must be witnessed by two registered nurses.

   Informed consents for non-English-speaking persons must be witnessed by one registered nurse, the name of the interpreter must be

FORM 1.1.1 continued

noted on the consent form, and the interpreter must sign the consent form.

The signatures of the patient or his or her health care surrogate or legitimate proxy on the form must attest to the following:

a. That the relevant health professional has explained to the patient, health care surrogate, or legitimate proxy in terms he or she is likely to understand

   i. The risks and benefits of the proposed treatment,

   ii. Alternative medical treatments available and their attendant risks,

   iii. The risks and medical consequences associated with the refusal of the contemplated treatment.

b. That the patient, health care surrogate, or legitimate proxy was given a reasonable opportunity to ask questions of the relevant health professionals and check his or her understanding of the proposed procedure.

c. That the patient, health care surrogate, or legitimate proxy is satisfied that procedures 1a and 1b have been adhered to.

2. If a patient is impaired in or lacks decision-making capacity, the patient's health care surrogate shall be notified and may give consent on behalf of the patient. If the patient has not designated a health care surrogate or the surrogate is not willing or able to perform his or her duties, a proxy must be notified and may give consent on behalf of the patient. The selection of a proxy shall be made in the following order of priority if no individual in a prior class is reasonably available, willing, or able to act:

a. The judicially appointed guardian who has been authorized to consent to medical treatment, if one has been previously appointed.

b. The patient's spouse.

c. An adult child of the patient or, if the patient has more than one adult child, a majority of the adult children who are reasonably available for consultation.

d. A parent of the patient.

FORM 1.1.1 continued

e. An adult sibling of the patient or, if the patient has more than one sibling, a majority of the adult siblings who are reasonably available for consultation.

f. An adult relative of the patient who has exhibited special care and concern for the patient, who has maintained regular contact with the patient, and who is familiar with the patient's activities, health, and religious or moral beliefs.

g. A close friend of the patient. The close friend must present an affidavit to the health care facility or the attending or treating physician stating that he or she is a friend of the patient, is willing and able to become involved in the patient's health care, and has maintained such regular contact with the patient as to be familiar with the patient's activities, health, religious or moral beliefs, and wishes regarding medical care. See **Form 3.3.2.**

If no individual in a prior class is reasonably available, willing, and competent to act, persons in the next priority class may decide.

Documentation of attempts to contact a health care surrogate or proxy should be indicated in the patient's medical record.

Except for minors who are emancipated, that is, those not under the custody of their parents; those who are married; those who are in the armed services; or those living independently, for all minors there shall be a legitimate proxy. The proxy shall be selected in the following order of priority:

a. The judicially appointed guardian of the patient if such guardian has been appointed and has been authorized to consent to medical treatment.

b. The natural or adoptive parents of the patient.

c. The nearest adult relative of the patient.

3. The informed consent is valid during the current hospital stay but can be revoked at any time by the selected proxy.

4. Where the patient lacks decision-making capacity for a valid informed consent and an investigation fails to reveal the presence of any health care surrogate, legal counsel will be contacted prior to the performance of any emergency medical treatment.

FORM 1.1.1 continued

5. Unless a surrogate or proxy has obtained court approval or a patient has expressly delegated authority to a surrogate or proxy, a surrogate or proxy may not provide consent for the following procedures:

   a. Abortion.

   b. Sterilization.

   c. Electroshock therapy.

   d. Psychosurgery.

   e. Experimental treatments or therapies that have not been approved by a federally approved institutional review board in compliance with 45 C.F.R, part 46, or 21 C.F.R., part 56.

   f. Voluntary admission to a mental health facility.

   g. Withholding or withdrawing life-prolonging procedures from a pregnant patient prior to viability of the fetus.

FORM 1.1.2
INFORMED CONSENT
FOR PROCEDURES AND OPERATIONS

Patient's name _____

Date _____

I hereby authorize Dr. _____
to perform on the above named patient the following described procedure or operation:

_____

_____

_____

_____

The general method of procedure or operation has been fully explained to me by the above named physician, who also explained to my satisfaction (1) the risks and benefits of the proposed procedure or operation; (2) the alternative medical treatments to the procedure or operation and their risks; (3) that one alternative was that I had the right to refuse the procedure or operation and the risks associated with refusal.

I was afforded full opportunity to ask the above named physician questions.

To advance medical education, I also consent to the presence of observers and the making of videotapes or the taking of photographs during the procedure or operation.

_____
Signature of patient

_____
Signature of health care surrogate or proxy if appropriate

_____
Signature of interpreter

_____
Signature of witness

FORM 1.1.3
CONSENT TO THE ADMINISTRATION OF ANESTHESIA

Patient's name_____

Date _____

I know that I will soon undergo the following described procedure or operation:

_____

_____

I consent to the administration of anesthetics by an anesthesiologist/anesthetist.

The administration of anesthesia and the common risks and alternatives have been explained to me by _____. He or she or other members of the ABC Hospital Department of Anesthesia will be responsible for my anesthetic care.

I understand that complications may arise as a result of the administration of anesthetics, such as allergic reactions, pneumonia, phlebitis, nerve injury or paralysis, broken teeth, or complications involving the heart, lungs, brain, liver, kidneys, nerves, and other organs. The psyche may be disordered. Death may result. If I am pregnant, the risks may affect the fetus. I acknowledge that no guarantees have been given as to the results and I assume the risk of anesthesia.

I also understand that the surgeons will be occupied only with the procedure or operation and that the determination, administration, and maintenance of anesthesia are the responsibility and function of the anesthesiologist/anesthetist. I understand also that several types of anesthesia may be used, including general anesthesia (sodium pentothal by injection or by inhalation agent), spinal anesthesia (such as saddle block), nerve block anesthesia, local anesthesia, or combinations of these types. The choice and any medically acceptable alternatives have been discussed with me by the anesthesiologist. I hereby consent to the administration of anesthesia by the following method:

_____

If, during the course of the procedure or operation, a condition arises that is unforeseen which calls for methods different from that now proposed, I hereby authorize and request the individual administering the anesthetic to do what he or she deems advisable under the circumstances.

FORM 1.1.3 continued

I have read this consent and understand and agree with its provisions. I was afforded full opportunity to ask the above named anesthesiologist/anesthetist questions and they were fully answered.

_____

Signature of patient

_____

Signature of health care surrogate or proxy if appropriate

_____

Signature of interpreter

_____

Signature of witness

_____

Signature of anesthesiologist

FORM 1.1.4
JEHOVAH'S WITNESS
REFUSAL OF BLOOD TRANSFUSION AND RELEASE

I, _____, date of birth, _____, am a member of the religious faith commonly known as the Jehovah's Witnesses and scrupulously follow the tenets and belief of that faith. It is my express understanding and belief that my faith does not allow the administration of blood transfusions of any kind for any purpose whatsoever. I therefore expressly refuse to allow anyone to administer a blood transfusion to me during the course of my hospitalization or during the _____procedure or surgery scheduled for me on _____at the ABC Hospital to be performed by Dr. _____.

The risks attendant upon my refusal to permit such a transfusion have been fully explained to me and I fully understand such risks. In addition, I fully understand that I will in all probability need a transfusion of blood or blood derivatives and that, if I do not allow such a transfusion, my chances for regaining normal health are seriously reduced. I also understand that in all probability my refusal to allow such treatment or procedures will seriously imperil my life and may possibly result in my death.

Even with this full understanding, I still refuse to give permission for such a transfusion of blood or blood derivatives as required for my safety or life, and I hereby release the hospital, any physicians connected with my care, and the nurses and employees of the hospital who have been or will be involved in the scheduled procedure or surgery from all liability for damages or injury to me or for my death for respecting and following my express wishes and directions on this matter. This release includes a full release from all manner of causes of action or suits which I now have or will have against the hospital or any physicians connected with my care by reason of the performance of the scheduled procedure or surgery.

_____   _____
Signature   Date

_____   _____
Witness   Date

_____   _____
Witness   Date

FORM 1.1.4 continued

I have explained in layman's language the implications of the above refusal
of blood and am satisfied that the patient understands his (her) actions.

Attending physician   Date

FORM 1.1.4.1
OPTIONAL CLAUSE WHERE PATIENT
WITH MINOR CHILDREN REFUSES BLOOD

If the patient has children below the age of eighteen whose health and welfare
have not been provided for, this form is void.

FORM 1.1.4.2
SECOND OPTIONAL CLAUSE WHERE PATIENT
WITH MINOR CHILDREN REFUSES BLOOD

If the patient has children below the age of eighteen whose health and welfare
have not been provided for, immediate notice is to be provided the state
attorney to allow the state attorney to take such action as is considered
appropriate for the protection of minor children.

FORM 1.1.5
REFUSAL OF BLOOD TRANSFUSION
(By Patient Who Is Not Jehovah's Witness)

I request that neither blood nor blood derivatives be administered to (patient's name)_____during this hospitalization. I hereby release the hospital, its personnel and agents, and all physicians connected with the patient's care from any responsibility whatsoever for unfavorable direct or indirect reactions or any untoward results due to my refusal to permit the use of blood or its derivatives. The possible consequences of such refusal on my part have been fully explained to me by my attending physician and I fully understand that such consequences, including the patient's death, may occur as a result of my refusal.

This release is binding upon myself and my heirs and representatives.

_____

Patient or legally authorized agent   Date

_____

Witness

_____

Witness

(One witness should be neither a spouse nor a blood relative of the patient.)

I have explained in layman's language the implications of the above refusal of blood and am satisfied that the patient or authorized agent understands his (her) actions.

_____

Attending physician   Date

FORM 1.2.1
REFUSAL OF MEDICAL TREATMENT AND RELEASE
BY PATIENT WITH DECISION-MAKING CAPACITY

(This form shall be void for minors [emancipated minors are treated as adults].)

I, _____ (patient), have been given relevant and essential information and an explanation by _____ (M.D./D.O.) regarding the nature of my condition; the purpose of the proposed treatment(s); the likely benefits, risks, and discomforts; and possible alternative medical treatment(s), including the option of no treatment, along with the risks, consequences, and benefits.

I, _____ (patient), nonetheless refuse to consent to the following medical treatment(s) because I view them as a heavy spiritual, psychological, physical, and/or economic burden either for myself or for those dear to me:

_____ Tubal feeding

_____ Mechanical respirator

_____ Dialysis

_____ Resuscitation (Coding)

_____ Transfusion of blood or blood products

_____ Other (specify) _____

I, _____ (patient), have been given the opportunity to ask questions and all my questions have been answered to my satisfaction.

The risks attendant upon my refusal have been fully explained to me, and I fully understand them and that in all probability my refusal will seriously imperil my health and may possibly result in my death.

I hereby release the hospital, any physicians connected with my care, and the nurses and employees of the hospital who have been or will be involved in my care from all liability and damages for injury to me or for my death for respecting my wishes and directions in this matter. This release includes a full release from all manner of causes of action or suits which I have or will have against the hospital or any physicians connected with my care by reason of respecting my wishes and directions.

FORM 1.2.1 continued

I confirm that I have read and fully understand the above prior to my own signing.

Signature   Date

Witness   Date

Witness   Date

(One witness should be neither the spouse nor a blood relative of the patient.)

I have explained in layman's language the implications of the above refusal and am satisfied that the patient understands his or her actions. The patient is able to acknowledge the presence of illness and verbalizes recognizable reasons(s) for his or her refusal of treatment(s) and understands the consequences of no treatment.

Attending physician   Date/Time

I have witnessed the attending physician's explanation and agree that the patient has chosen to refuse treatment(s), understands the relevant information, appreciates the situation and its consequences, and can explain the basis for his or her refusal.

Witness   Date

Interpreter   Date

FORM 1.3.1
HOSPITAL POLICY AND PROCEDURES—
REFUSAL OF TREATMENT BY PATIENTS WITH
DECISION-MAKING CAPACITY AND BY PATIENTS
WITHOUT DECISION-MAKING CAPACITY

POLICY

1. This hospital recognizes the right to patient autonomy, that is, for a patient to participate in decisions affecting his or her life and to have his or her wishes respected, within the law. Patients with decision-making capacity have the right to refuse all care and procedures whether they are life-sustaining or routine.

2. A health care surrogate or legitimate proxy may refuse treatment for patients who are neither terminal nor vegetative and who lack decision-making capacity.

3. If possible, efforts should be made to correct the impairment in capacity. If it is not corrected, treatment decisions by a health care surrogate or proxy shall be based on the substituted judgment standard and his or her reasonable belief that the patient would make the same decision if the patient had decision-making capacity. Generally, decisions of the health care surrogate should be in accordance with written or oral advance directives. Decisions by proxies should be in accordance with the patient's views about medical treatment for the patient, the patient's previous statements about the medical care administered to others, or the patient's religious beliefs.

4. For those patients who lack decision-making capacity, in the absence of a health care surrogate or legitimate proxy, treatment shall be provided. If treatment appears futile based on medical facts, then the health team is referred to the policy Withholding and Withdrawing Life-Sustaining Procedures from Adult Terminally Ill Patients (Form 4.2.1).

5. In an emergency or life-threatening situation, when there is substantial evidence of the impairment of the patient's decision-making capacity in the absence of a health care surrogate or proxy, the attending/admitting/treating physician may override the patient's refusal of treatment and implement medical treatment. When the patient's condition permits, the physician may request further evaluation of the patient's decision-making capacity. After further evaluation, efforts will be made to contact a health care surrogate or proxy for future health care decisions.

FORM 1.3.1 continued

PROCEDURE FOR A PATIENT WITH
DECISION-MAKING CAPACITY

1. The attending physician shall communicate to the patient the information pertinent to a specific decision in terms her or she is likely to understand, that is, the nature of his or her condition and the proposed intervention; the likely benefits, risks, and discomforts; and possible alternatives, including the option of no treatment, along with the risks, consequences, benefits, and possible complications in the recovery process.

2. Another person shall witness the physician's explanation. The witness shall attest, by signature, that the patient has made a decision, understands the relevant information, appreciates the situation and its consequences, and can explain the basis for his or her refusal.

3. The patient's refusal of medical treatment should be honored by the attending physician.

4. Evaluation of patient's decision-making capacity by the attending physician shall be documented in the medical records.

5. The nursing administration shall be notified.

6. The patient shall complete a Refusal of Medical Treatment and Release form (**Form 1.2.1**). Note: This form shall be void for minors (emancipated minors are treated as adults).

PROCEDURE FOR A PATIENT WHO LACKS
DECISION-MAKING CAPACITY

1. When a patient's capacity to make his or her own health care decisions or to provide informed consent is in question, the following procedure is to be followed:

   a. The attending physician shall evaluate the patient's capacity and document that evaluation in the patient's medical record.

   b. If the attending physician concludes that the patient lacks capacity, the hospital shall have another physician, not employed by the hospital or associated with the attending physician, evaluate the patient's capacity.

   c. If the second physician agrees that the patient lacks capacity, his or her evaluation shall also be documented in the patient's record.

FORM 1.3.1 continued

2. If a patient is impaired in or lacks decision-making capacity, the patient's health care surrogate shall be notified to make health care decisions consistent with a patient's advance directive. If the patient has not designated a health care surrogate or the surrogate is not willing or able to perform his or her duties, a proxy must be notified to make health care decisions based on the subjective standard. The selection of a proxy shall be made in the following order of priority if no individual in a prior class is reasonably available, willing, or competent to act:

   a. The judicially appointed guardian of the patient authorized to consent to medical treatment, if such a guardian has been appointed. This paragraph shall not be construed to require such appointment before a decision can be made.

   b. The patient's spouse.

   c. An adult child of the patient or, if the patient has more than one adult child, a majority of the adult children who are reasonably available for consultation.

   d. A parent of the patient.

   e. An adult sibling of the patient or, if the patient has more than one sibling, a majority of the adult siblings who are reasonably available for consultation.

   f. An adult relative of the patient who has exhibited special care and concern for the patient, who has maintained regular contact with the patient, and who is familiar with the patient's activities, health, and religious or moral beliefs.

   g. A close friend of the patient.

   In the case of minors, the selection of a legitimate proxy shall involve the following order of priority:

   a. The judicially appointed guardian of the patient if such guardian has been appointed.

   b. The parents of the patient.

   c. The nearest adult relative of the patient.

3. A witness should be present when the attending physician explains to the health care surrogate or legitimate proxy (in terms the surrogate or proxy is likely to understand) the reasons for treatment

FORM 1.3.1 continued

and the risks or consequences of refusing treatment. The proxy should be able to explain the basis for his or her refusal.

4. Another person shall witness the physician's explanation. The witness shall attest, by signature, that the patient has made a decision, understands the relevant information, appreciates the situation and its consequences, and can explain the basis for his or her refusal.

5. The attending physician and two other physicians shall include statements in the progress notes on the following:

   a. The patient's condition and level of mental and physical function.

   b. The degree of pain and discomfort currently being experienced by the patient and the degree expected in the future.

   c. The nature of the medical treatment to be withheld or withdrawn including benefits, risks, invasiveness, painfulness, and side effects.

   d. The patient's prognosis without medical assistance.

   e. The physicians' belief of the appropriateness of removing or withdrawing the proposed treatment within medical ethics.

   f. The physicians' determination of whether there is any reasonable probability that the patient will regain decision-making capacity.

6. For refusal of cardiopulmonary resuscitative measures, see the Do-Not-Resuscitate Order Policy (**Form 5.2.1 or 5.2.1.3**).

7. The surrogate's or legitimate proxy's decision is to be based on the subjective standard. The surrogate's or proxy's refusal of treatment for a patient lacking in decision-making capacity shall be honored by this hospital and the attending physician.

8. Have surrogate or proxy complete a Refusal of Medical Treatment and Release form (**Form 1.3.4**).

9. Notify nursing administration.

FORM 1.3.1.1
OPTIONAL CLAUSE
TO EXPEDITE GUARDIANSHIP PROCEEDINGS

In the event a patient lacks decision-making capacity or has not designated a surrogate and it appears that no individuals authorized to act as legitimate proxies for the patient will or can be found, the social services department will be contacted immediately to expedite procedures for the appointment of a guardian authorized to make health care decisions.

FORM 1.3.1.2
OPTIONAL PREGNANCY CLAUSE

The refusal of treatment by a pregnant patient shall be void.

FORM 1.3.2
NOTIFICATION TO HEALTH CARE SURROGATE

Surrogate's name _____

Address _____

Please be advised that_____, who is a patient in the ABC Hospital, designated you as health care surrogate to make health care decisions on the patient's behalf in case the patient was not able to make these decisions.

Since two physicians have agreed that the patient lacks the capacity to make decisions, your authority as surrogate has begun.

If you require further information, please communicate with our social services department at extension_____.

FORM 1.3.3
NOTIFICATION TO PROXY

Proxy's name _____

Address _____

Please be advised that_____is a patient in the ABC Hospital. This patient has not designated a health care surrogate to make health care decisions on the patient's behalf in case the patient was not able to make these decisions.

Since two physicians have agreed that the patient lacks the capacity to make decisions and your relationship to the patient is_____, your authority as proxy has begun.

If you require further information, please communicate with our social services department at extension_____.

FORM 1.3.4
SURROGATE'S, GUARDIAN'S, OR PROXY'S
REFUSAL OF MEDICAL TREATMENT AND RELEASE

Re: Patient _____

I,_____, certify
that I am authorized to provide refusal of treatment on behalf of the above
named patient by virtue of my relationship to the patient as (health care
surrogate, court-appointed guardian, or legitimate proxy). I have been
given relevant and essential information and an explanation by
_____ (M.D./D.O.) regarding the nature
of the patient's condition; the purpose of the proposed treatment(s); the likely
benefits, risks, and discomforts; and possible alternative medical treatment(s),
including the option of no treatment, along with the risks, consequences, and
benefits.

Nonetheless, based on my reasonable belief that the patient would make this
same decision had the patient been capable, I refuse on behalf of the patient
to consent to the following medical treatment(s):

_____ Tubal feeding

_____ Mechanical respirator

_____ Dialysis

_____ Resuscitation (Coding)

_____ Transfusion of blood or blood products

_____ Other (specify) _____

I have been given the opportunity to ask questions and all my questions have
been answered to my satisfaction.

The risks attendant upon my refusal have been fully explained to me, and I
fully understand them and that in all probability my refusal will seriously
imperil the patient's health and may possibly result in his or her death.

I hereby release the hospital, any physicians connected with the patient's care,
and the nurses and employees of the hospital who have been or will be
involved in his or her care from all liability and damages for injury to him or
her or for his or her death for respecting his or her or my wishes and directions
in this matter. This release includes a full release from all manner of causes
of action or suits which the patient or I have or will have against the hospital

FORM 1.3.4 continued

or any physicians connected with the patient's care by reason of respecting his or her or my wishes and directions.

I confirm that I have read and fully understand the above prior to my own signing.

_____

Signature of surrogate or guardian or proxy   Date

_____

Witness   Date

_____

Witness   Date

I have explained in layman's language the implications of the above refusal and am satisfied that the surrogate or legitimate proxy understands his or her actions. The surrogate, guardian, or legitimate proxy is able to acknowledge the presence of illness and to verbalize the recognizable reason(s) for his or her refusal of treatment(s) and understands the consequences of no treatment.

_____

Attending physician   Date/Time

I have witnessed the attending physician's explanation and agree that the surrogate, guardian, or legitimate proxy has chosen to refuse treatment(s), understands the relevant information, appreciates the situation and its consequences, and can explain the basis for his or her refusal.

_____

Witness   Date

_____

Interpreter   Date

FORM 1.9.1
RELEASE BY PATIENT LEAVING HOSPITAL AGAINST MEDICAL ADVICE

Patient _____

Date _____

This is to certify that, against the advice of the authorities at the ABC Hospital and my attending physician, it is my wish to leave the ABC Hospital at this time. I have made this decision on my own volition after having had fully explained to me the risks attendant upon my decision to leave the hospital prematurely. I hereby release the hospital and my attending physician and the nurses and employees of the hospital who have been involved with my care from all liability in this matter.

_____

Signature

I hereby agree to indemnify and save harmless from all liability as a result of the discharge of the patient the ABC Hospital, the patient's attending physician, and the nurses and employees of the ABC Hospital who have been involved in the patient's care.

_____

Spouse, parent, or other relation

FORM 2.3.1
LIVING WILLS: QUESTIONS AND ANSWERS

What are living wills?

They are written directives executed and witnessed like a will which are recognized as valid by the several statutes known as "natural death" or "living will" laws. They need not be prepared by an attorney. They permit competent adults to express their wishes about implementing, withholding, or withdrawing life-sustaining medical treatment in the event they are terminally ill.

Are living wills necessary?

You have the right to control decisions regarding life-sustaining medical care. But you may lose your ability to express your wishes. Living wills are the means of expressing your wishes in advance of this loss of ability, of preserving your autonomy, and of relieving your family and physician of a painful burden.

If you can't express your wishes about your own medical care, can another person make medical decisions for you?

The living will allows you to appoint someone else to make medical decisions in line with your wishes.

Must a living will be witnessed?

Two adults must witness the will when you sign it. But one witness should not be your spouse or blood relative.

After you have signed a living will, who should receive copies of it?

To be sure that your wishes are carried out, it is vital that others know that you have made a living will. So a copy should be given to your physician and your next of kin. Copies may also be given to your attorney and religious advisor.

Does making a living will affect life insurance?

Your existing life insurance policies are not invalidated, and you cannot be turned down by an insurance company, if you have made a living will.

If you refuse life-sustaining procedures in a living will, does this amount to committing suicide?

No, it does not because it is not your refusal of treatment that causes your death but an underlying disease or condition.

FORM 2.3.1 continued

After you make a living will, can you change it or revoke it?

The wording can always be altered and additional directions given. If you decide that you do not want a living will, it can always be revoked.

Are a living trust and a living will the same?

A living trust deals with assets, not with medical treatment. It is not the same as a living will.

Do physicians approve of living wills?

The great majority of doctors support them.

Should you discuss the provisions of a living will with your doctor?

Yes, you should ask your doctor to talk with you about what medical treatment you will need if you are seriously ill.

FORM 2.3.2
LIVING WILL
(Evaluation of Condition by One Physician)

To my family, physicians, and all those concerned with my care:

Declaration made this ___day of_____, 19___.

I,_____,
voluntarily and willfully make known my desire that my dying not be artificially prolonged under the circumstances set forth below and I do hereby declare:

If at any time I have a terminal condition and if my attending or treating physician has determined that there is no medical probability of my recovery from such condition, I direct that life-sustaining procedures be withheld or withdrawn when the application of such procedures would serve only to prolong artificially the process of dying, and that I be permitted to die naturally with only the administration of medication or the performance of any medical procedure deemed necessary to provide me with comfort care or to alleviate pain.

It is my intention that this declaration be honored by my family and physician as the final expression of my legal rights to refuse medical or surgical treatment and to accept the consequences of such refusal.

I understand the full import of this declaration and I am emotionally and mentally competent to make this declaration.

_____

Signature

_____

Witness

_____

Address   Phone

_____

Witness

_____

Address   Phone

FORM 2.3.3
LIVING WILL
(Evaluation of Condition by Two Physicians)

To my family, physicians, and all those concerned with my care:

Declaration made this ___day of_____, 19___.

I, _____,
voluntarily and willfully make known my desire that my dying not be artificially prolonged under the circumstances set forth below and I do hereby declare:

If at any time I have a terminal condition and if my attending or treating physician and another consulting physician have determined that there is no medical probability of my recovery from such condition, I direct that life-sustaining procedures be withheld or withdrawn when the application of such procedures would serve only to prolong artificially the process of dying, and that I be permitted to die naturally with only the administration of medication or the performance of any medical procedure deemed necessary to provide me with comfort care or to alleviate pain.

It is my intention that this declaration be honored by my family and physician as the final expression of my legal rights to refuse medical or surgical treatment and to accept the consequences of such refusal.

I understand the full import of this declaration and I am emotionally and mentally competent to make this declaration.

_____
Signature

_____
Witness

_____
Address   Phone

_____
Witness

_____
Address   Phone

FORM 2.3.4
DIRECTION CONCERNING THE WITHHOLDING
OR WITHDRAWING OF ARTIFICIAL FEEDING

I do__do not__ desire that nutrition and hydration (food and water) be withheld or withdrawn when artificially or technologically supplied nutrition or hydration would serve only to prolong artificially the process of dying.

FORM 2.3.5
ADDITIONAL INSTRUCTIONS

Additional instructions (optional):

_____

_____

_____

_____

FORM 2.3.6
OPTIONAL PREGNANCY CLAUSE

If I have been diagnosed as pregnant and that diagnosis is known to my physician, this living will shall have no effect during the course of my pregnancy.

FORM 2.3.7
DIRECTION CONCERNING
TERMINATION OF LIFE SUPPORT IF PREGNANT

Should I be pregnant, I__do __do not confer on my surrogate the authority to provide consent for the withholding or withdrawing of life-sustaining treatment prior to the viability of my fetus.

FORM 2.3.8
REVOCATION

I hereby revoke my Living Will Declaration dated the ____day of _____, 19____.

Date _____

_____

Declarant

FORM 3.2.1
ADVANCE DIRECTIVES: QUESTIONS AND ANSWERS

What is an advance directive?

It is a written or oral instruction you may give before you are seriously ill about future medical treatment or an appointment you may make of an individual to make decisions about this treatment if you cannot make them. The advance directive permits the individual to control decisions regarding his or her medical treatment.

What kinds of advance directives are there?

There are three kinds: the living will, the health care surrogate designation, and the durable power of attorney for health care.

Is an advance directive only for elderly people?

No. At any time of life, a person may lose the ability to express his or her wishes and choices regarding medical treatment. Any individual who believes that these wishes and choices should be honored should make any of the above kinds of advance directives.

Does the law require you to make an advance directive?

No. But if you have not made an advance directive and are unable to make your own health care decisions, the law permits decisions to be made for you by a proxy, that is, a guardian appointed by a court, your spouse, adult child, parent, adult brother or sister, adult relative, or close friend.

Must an advance directive be prepared by a lawyer?

It is not necessary for a lawyer to be consulted by the majority of people who complete advance directives. But if there is something in an advance directive that is not understood, lawyer's advice may be needed.

Where can you get free forms of advance directives?

Advance directive forms are generally available in the admitting offices of hospitals, or you may ask a hospital social worker or request them from your physician. Several organizations provide them as well. Choice in Dying distributes free state-specific advance directives. Their toll-free number is 800–989–WILL, and their address is 200 Varick St., New York, NY 10014. There is also the Legal Hotline for Older Americans, P.O. Box 23810, Pittsburgh, PA 15222 (1–800–262–5297) and Legal Counsel for the Elderly (associated with the American Association for Retired Persons), 1331 H Street, Washington, DC 20005 (202–434–2120). In addition, some state

FORM 3.2.1 continued

and local bar associations, state medical associations, state offices for the aging, and state and voluntary hospital associations may provide forms. You may use their forms and change any of the words you wish and add any further instructions.

Where can you get free legal information?

There are several organizations that will provide free information. One is Choice in Dying, a national nonprofit organization in New York, which has a toll-free information hotline (given above).

For how long is the advance directive good?

It remains valid until you cancel or change it in writing or orally. If you do not cancel or change it, it is a good idea to update it from time to time to show that it is still something you want.

FORM 3.2.2
LIVING WILL DESIGNATION OF SURROGATE

In the event that I have been determined to be unable to provide express and informed consent regarding the withholding, withdrawing, or continuing of life-sustaining procedures, I wish to designate as my surrogate to carry out the provisions of this declaration:

Name _____

Address _____

Phone _____

FORM 3.2.3
ADVISORY FOR PATIENTS
ABOUT HEALTH CARE SURROGATE DESIGNATIONS

Your health care surrogate designation lets you name a person who will make health care decisions for you in case you do not have the ability to make them yourself.

These decisions can be made for you whenever you cannot speak for yourself, not only when you are terminally ill.

The individual you designate should be a person in whom you have confidence, with whom you have talked about your wishes and beliefs, and who will accept responsibility for carrying out your wishes and making decisions on your behalf.

The form does not have to be prepared by a lawyer or be notarized. You must sign it and two witnesses must sign it also. One of the witnesses must not be your spouse or a blood relative. The surrogate cannot sign as a witness.

A copy of the form must be given to your surrogate, and other copies should be given to your physician and family.

FORM 3.2.4
HEALTH CARE SURROGATE DESIGNATION

In the event that I have been determined to be incapacitated to provide informed consent for medical treatment and surgical and diagnostic procedures, I wish to designate as my surrogate for health care decisions:

Name_____

Address_____

Phone_____

If my surrogate is unwilling or unable to perform the surrogate's duties, I wish to designate as my alternate surrogate:

Name_____

Address_____

Phone_____

I fully understand that this designation will permit my designee to make health care decisions and to provide, withhold, or withdraw consent on my behalf; to apply for public benefits to defray the cost of health care; and to authorize my admission to or transfer from a health care facility.

Additional instructions (optional): _____

_____

_____

I further affirm that this designation is not being made as a condition of treatment or admission to a health facility. I will notify and send a copy of this document to the following persons other than my surrogate so they may know who my surrogate is:

Name_____

Name_____

_____
Signature   Date

Witness _____

Witness _____

FORM 3.2.4.1
ALTERNATE HEALTH CARE SURROGATE DESIGNATION

In the event that I have been determined to be incapacitated to provide informed consent for medical treatment and surgical and diagnostic procedures, I wish to designate as my surrogate for health care decisions:

Name _____

Address _____

Phone _____

If my surrogate is unwilling or unable to perform the surrogate's duties, I wish to designate as my alternate surrogate:

Name _____

Address _____

Phone _____

I fully understand that this designation will permit my designee to make health care decisions and to provide, withhold, or withdraw consent on my behalf; to apply for public benefits to defray the cost of health care; and to authorize my admission to or transfer from a health care facility.

Withholding or withdrawing life-sustaining procedures: __I do__I do not authorize my surrogate to consent to the withholding or withdrawal of life-sustaining procedures if I am terminally ill and I lack decision-making capacity with no reasonable medical probability of recovering such capacity.

Additional instructions (optional):_____

_____

_____

I further affirm that this designation is not being made as a condition of treatment or admission to a health facility.

_____
Signature   Date

Witness _____

Witness _____

FORM 3.2.4.2
SECOND ALTERNATE
HEALTH CARE SURROGATE DESIGNATION

I,_____, do hereby
designate_____ to serve as my health care
surrogate in the event that I have been determined to be incapacitated to
provide informed consent for medical treatment.

_____

Signature   Date

Witness _____

Witness _____

FORM 3.2.5
DURABLE POWER OF ATTORNEY FOR HEALTH CARE

I, _____,
do hereby appoint_____, whose address
is _____ and whose relationship to me
is_____, my true and lawful agent and attorney-in-fact granting to him or her full power and authority to make any and all health care
decisions for me should I become unable to make my own health care
decisions. This appointment gives my agent the power to grant, refuse, or
withdraw consent on my behalf for any health care service, treatment, or
medical, therapeutic, or surgical procedure, including but not limited to
decisions regarding the withholding or withdrawing of life-sustaining treatment and do-not-resuscitate orders.

This durable power of attorney shall be effective if and when I become
incapable of making my own health care decisions and shall not be affected
by my disability. This durable power of attorney is nondelegable and shall be
valid until I die, revoke it, or am adjudged incompetent by a court.

IN WITNESS WHEREOF, I have set my hand and seal this ____day of
_____, 199__.

Principal _____

Witness _____

Address _____

Witness _____

Address _____

State of _____ County of _____

BE IT KNOWN that on the __day of_____, 199__, before me personally
appeared_____, to me known to be the person described in
and who executed this durable power of attorney, and he/she acknowledged
to me that he/she executed said instrument freely and for the purposes therein
mentioned.

IN TESTIMONY WHEREOF, I have hereunto subscribed my name and
affixed my seal of office the day and year above written.

_____

Notary public, state of _____My commission expires: _____

FORM 3.2.5.1
ALTERNATE GENERAL
AND HEALTH CARE DURABLE POWER OF ATTORNEY

Know all men by these presents that I, _____,
hereby appoint_____, whose address
is_____ and whose relation to me is
_____, my true and lawful attorney-in-fact for me and
in my name, place, and stead, giving and granting unto my attorney-in-fact
full power and authority to perform any and all acts and do things of every
kind and nature that should be performed or done in the management of my
own personal life and business affairs, as I might or could do if personally
present, hereby ratifying and confirming all that my attorney-in-fact shall
lawfully do or cause to be done by virtue hereof.

This power includes the authority to obtain and release my medical records,
claim medical benefits to which I may be entitled, and arrange for and consent
to medical care, including medical, diagnostic, therapeutical, and surgical
procedures; the administration of medications and drugs; and the use of
mechanical or other procedures relating to bodily functions including but
not limited to artificial feeding, artificial respiration, and cardiopulmonary
resuscitation.

This durable power of attorney is nondelegable and shall not be affected by
my disability except as provided by statute. It is valid until I die, revoke the
power, or am adjudged by a court as being incompetent. In the event a
petition to determine my competency or appoint a guardian for me has been
filed, this power of attorney shall be temporarily suspended until the petition
is dismissed or withdrawn or I am adjudged competent, at which time this
power shall be automatically reinstated and any exercise of it shall be valid.
If I am adjudged incompetent, this power shall be automatically revoked.

IN WITNESS WHEREOF, I have set my hand and seal this ____day of
_____, 199__.

Principal _____

Witness _____

Address_____

Witness _____

Address_____

FORM 3.2.5.1 continued

State of _____ County of _____

BE IT KNOWN that on the ___day of_____, 199__, before me personally appeared_____, to me known to be the person described in and who executed this durable power of attorney, and he/she acknowledged to me that he/she executed said instrument freely and for the purposes therein mentioned.

IN TESTIMONY WHEREOF, I have hereunto subscribed my name and affixed my seal of office the day and year above written.

_____

Notary public, state of _____My commission expires: _____

FORM 3.2.5.2
OPTIONAL CLAUSE
TO DETERMINE PRINCIPAL'S INCAPACITY

This durable power of attorney shall become effective when I do not have the capacity to manage my affairs as determined by statements in writing from my spouse and lawyer retained by me prior to my incapacity.

FORM 3.2.5.3
SECOND OPTIONAL CLAUSE
TO DETERMINE PRINCIPAL'S INCAPACITY

This durable power of attorney is nondelegable and shall not be affected by my disability except as provided by law. It shall become effective when my attending physician and a consulting physician certify that I do not have decision-making capacity for the purpose of giving informed consent for health care decisions.

FORM 3.2.6
ADVANCE DIRECTIVE CARD FOR HEALTH PROVIDERS

To my health providers:

My name is _____ .

The following advance directives have been completed by me:

_____ Living will

_____ Health care surrogate designation

_____ Durable power of attorney for health care

_____ Other _____

These directives can be found in_____ .

I have designated the following person as my surrogate or agent:

Name_____

Address_____

Phone_____

_____

Signature   Date

FORM 3.3.1
HOSPITAL POLICY AND PROCEDURES—
PATIENTS WITH ADVANCE DIRECTIVES

POLICY

This hospital recognizes its responsibility under the Patient Self-Determination Act to maintain a policy and procedures respecting advance directives.

It also recognizes the right of a competent individual of at least eighteen years of age to make an advance directive. *Advance directive* means a written witnessed document or oral statement in which instructions are given by a principal or in which a principal's desires are expressed concerning any aspect of the principal's health care.

In this policy an advance directive includes a living will or declaration, a durable power of attorney, and a health care surrogate designation.

PROCEDURES

I. GENERAL

A. An advance directive should be reviewed to determine that it complies with the requirements of the state's law.

B. If an advance directive is executed in language other than English, the advance directive shall be interpreted by a qualified interpreter familiar with the language in which the advance directive is executed. The name of the interpreter shall be documented in the patient's medical record.

C. Patients shall be provided with written information concerning their rights to make advance directives and this hospital's policies regarding such rights.

D. Whether or not an individual has made an advance directive shall be documented in the patient's medical record.

II. LIVING WILLS OR DECLARATIONS

A. Written declarations: In order to be a valid declaration, a living will or advance directive regarding the withholding or withdrawing of life-prolonging procedures must meet the following requirements. The document must:

1. Be in writing.

FORM 3.3.1 continued

2. Be signed by an adult declarant in the presence of two subscribing witnesses, one of whom is neither a spouse or a blood relative of the declarant.

B. Oral declarations: An oral declaration may only be given if the declarant is physically unable to sign a written declaration, and subsequent to the time the patient is diagnosed as suffering from a terminal condition.

In order to be a valid oral declaration, the declaration must:

1. Be reduced to writing.

2. Be given by the declarant in the presence of two subscribing witnesses, one of whom is neither a spouse nor a blood relative of the declarant.

3. Have the declarant's signature subscribed thereon by one of the subscribing witnesses who signed such declaration for the declarant while in the declarant's presence and at the declarant's direction.

C. It shall be the responsibility of the declarant to provide for notification to his or her attending physician that an advance directive has been made. The attending physician shall promptly document the advance directive in the patient's medical record. In the event that the declarant is comatose, incompetent, or otherwise mentally or physically incapable, any other person may notify the attending physician of the existence of an advance directive. If the advance directive is oral, the attending physician shall promptly make the fact of such advance directive a part of the patient's medical record.

D. Revocation: A declaration may be revoked at any time by the declarant:

1. By means of a signed, dated writing.

2. By means of the physical cancellation or destruction of the declaration by the declarant or by another in the declarant's presence and at the declarant's direction.

3. By means of an oral expression of an intent to revoke.

Any such revocation will be effective when it is communicated to the attending physician. No civil or criminal liability shall be

FORM 3.3.1 continued

imposed upon any person for failure to act upon a revocation unless the person has actual knowledge of such revocation.

If the hospital staff becomes aware of a patient's oral expression of intent to revoke a declaration, the declaration is revoked and such information shall be documented in the patient's medical record. Furthermore, the provisions of such a revoked declaration shall not be effective or followed by hospital staff.

III. DURABLE POWER OF ATTORNEY

A durable power of attorney is an instrument that is executed by a principal who authorizes someone to manage his or her affairs or make medical treatment decisions. To be valid, it must:

- be in writing,
- be signed by one or more witnesses, and
- contain the words "This durable power of attorney shall not be affected by the disability of the principal except as provided by statute."

It is no longer valid if the principal:

- dies,
- revokes the power, or
- is determined by a court as incompetent.

If it is invalid, the person named in it has no authority to act for the principal. Hospital staff members should ascertain from the person named in the power whether any of the just-named facts exist which would make the power invalid. The person is to make an affidavit stating whether or not such facts exist and the same shall be placed in the medical record.

IV. HEALTH CARE SURROGATE DESIGNATION

A. A health care surrogate designation authorizes a competent adult to make health care decisions for the patient upon the patient's incapacity. For it to be valid, the following requirements must be met:

1. The designation must be a written document.

Form 3.3.1 continued

2. It must be signed by the patient (designator); or in case of a patient unable to sign, the patient, in the presence of witnesses, must direct another person to sign the patient's name.

3. The signature must be made or acknowledged by the patient in the presence of two adult attesting witnesses.

4. The designated surrogate shall not act as a witness, and at least one witness shall not be the patient's spouse or blood relative.

B. The designation remains valid until revoked or terminates when a time specified in it expires.

When a patient's capacity to make his or her own health care decisions or to provide informed consent is in question, the following procedure is to be followed:

1. The attending physician shall evaluate the patient's capacity and document that evaluation in the patient's medical record.

2. If the attending physician concludes that the patient lacks capacity, the hospital shall have another physician, not employed by the hospital or associated with the attending physician, evaluate the patient's capacity.

3. If the second physician agrees that the patient lacks capacity, his or her evaluation shall also be documented in the patient's record.

4. If the patient lacks capacity and has designated a health care surrogate, the surrogate shall be given written notice that his or her authority has begun.

5. If the patient has designated an alternate surrogate and the original surrogate is unwilling or unable to perform his or her duties, the alternate surrogate shall be given written notice that his or her authority has begun.

6. If neither the original nor the alternate surrogate is able or willing to perform their duties, the hospital is to seek the appointment of a proxy in the following order of precedence:

   a. The judicially appointed guardian who has been authorized to consent to medical treatment, if one has been previously appointed.

   b. The patient's spouse.

FORM 3.3.1 continued

c. An adult child of the patient, or if the patient has more than one adult child, a majority of the adult children who are reasonably available for consultation.

d. A parent of the patient.

e. An adult sibling of the patient, or if the patient has more than one sibling, a majority of the adult siblings who are reasonably available for consultation.

f. An adult relative of the patient who has exhibited special care and concern for the patient, who has maintained regular contact with the patient, and who is familiar with the patient's activities, health, and religious or moral beliefs.

g. A close friend of the patient. The close friend must present an affidavit to the health care facility or the attending or treating physician stating that he or she is a friend of the patient, is willing and able to become involved in the patient's health care, and has maintained such regular contact with the patient as to be familiar with the patient's activities, health, religious or moral beliefs, and wishes regarding medical care. See **Form 3.3.2.**

If no individual in a prior class is reasonably available, willing, and competent to act, persons in the next priority class may decide.

Documentation of attempts to contact a health care surrogate or proxy should be indicated in the patient's medical record.

D. Authority and restrictions: Health care surrogates shall:

1. Have final authority to act for the patient and to make health care decisions for the patient during the patient's incapacity, unless the designation provides otherwise.

2. Consult with appropriate health care providers to provide informed consent in the best interests of the patient and make health care decisions for the patient which the surrogate believes the patient would have made under the circumstances if the patient were capable of making such decisions.

3. Give consent for medical or surgical treatment in writing using the appropriate consent forms.

FORM 3.3.1 continued

4. Have access to appropriate clinical records of the patient and have authority to authorize the release of information and clinical records to appropriate persons to ensure the continuity of the patient's health care.

5. Apply for public benefits, such as Medicare and Medicaid, for the patient and have access to information regarding the patient's income and assets to the extent required to make application. The hospital may not make such application a condition of continued care if the patient, if capable, would have refused to apply.

6. Authorize the transfer and admission of the patient to or from the hospital.

Unless a patient has specifically delegated written authority to a surrogate or a proxy or the surrogate or proxy has obtained judicial approval, the surrogate or proxy cannot consent to abortion, electroshock therapy, psychosurgery, experimental treatment not recommended by a federally approved institutional review board, voluntary admission to a mental health facility, or the withholding or withdrawing of life-sustaining treatment from a pregnant patient prior to the viability of the fetus.

E. Judicial review: The staff of the hospital, attending physician, or patient or patient's family may ask for judicial review of the decision of a proxy or surrogate if the individual believes that:

- the surrogate or proxy was not properly designated
- the designation of the surrogate is not effective any longer
- the decision was not in accord with the patient's known desires
- the patient changed his or her mind after it was executed

F. Revocation: Unless it expressly provides otherwise, the designation of a health care surrogate revokes any prior designations.

During a patient's stay at the hospital, the attending physician and the health care surrogate shall review the patient's capacity to consent: (1) every 30 days or (2) at any time requested by the patient. This review shall be documented in the patient's medical record.

If the patient requests the revocation of his or her designation of a health care surrogate, the attending physician shall evaluate the

FORM 3.3.1 continued

patient's capacity, and the hospital shall have another physician, not employed by the hospital or associated with the attending physician, evaluate the patient's capacity. The patient's request and both evaluations of the patient's capacity shall be documented in the patient's medical record. If both physicians agree that the patient has regained the capacity to make his or her own health care decisions and to provide informed consent, the appointment of a health care surrogate is revoked, and the patient's own health care decisions shall be followed.

Unless the designation expressly provides otherwise, if a patient has designated his or her spouse as health care surrogate, the subsequent dissolution or annulment of the marriage of the patient automatically revokes the designation of a patient's spouse as health care surrogate.

FORM 3.3.2
AFFIDAVIT OF CLOSE PERSONAL FRIEND

State of _____ County of_____

Before me, the undersigned authority, personally appeared_____
_____, whose address is
_____, who after being duly sworn
on oath deposes and says:

1. I am at least eighteen years of age, competent, and under no disability.

2. I am and have been a close personal friend of the patient _____ with whom I have maintained regular contact for___(months) (years) and am familiar with the patient's activities, health, and religious and moral beliefs.

3. I am willing and able to become involved in the patient's health care.

Further affiant sayeth not.

_____

Friend's signature

State of _____ County of_____

The foregoing instrument was acknowledged before me this__day of _____, 199__, by _____, who is personally known to me or who produced _____ as identification and who did take an oath.

IN TESTIMONY WHEREOF, I have hereunto subscribed my name and affixed my seal of office the day and year above written.

_____

Notary public, state of _____My commission expires: _____

FORM 3.4.1
CERTIFICATION OF ADULT TERMINAL CONDITION AND DECISION-MAKING CAPACITY

Patient's name _____

Terminal Condition

We certify that the above patient has a terminal condition.

Terminal means (please check condition corresponding to patient diagnosis):

____1. A condition caused by injury, disease, or illness for which there is no reasonable probability of recovery and which, without treatment, can be expected to cause death.

____2. A persistent vegetative state characterized by a permanent and irreversible condition of unconsciousness in which there is

   a. The absence of voluntary action or cognitive behavior of any kind, and

   b. An inability to communicate or interact purposefully with the environment.

____3. The patient has existed in such condition for at least a period of ____months because of (check one):

   a. hypoxia-ischemia

   b. closed head injury

   c. other etiology (please list): _____.

____4. There has been no improvement since this assessment for a period of at least __months.

Decision-Making Capacity

Patients with decision-making capacity can (1) make a decision; (2) understand the relevant information (including paraphrasing in the patient's own words what a health care provider has explained); (3) appreciate the situation and its consequences; and (4)can explain the basis for consent or refusal.

This patient ____does____does not have decision-making capacity for the purpose of providing informed consent for a health care decision.

FORM 3.4.1 continued

Documentation of Patient Assessment

We have examined the above named patient and have documented in the patient's medical record the objective criteria according to which we have made our assessments concerning the patient's terminal condition and decision-making capacity.

Patient's attending physician   Date

Patient's consulting physician   Date

FORM 4.1.1
DESIGNEE'S AGREEMENT TO WITHHOLD
OR WITHDRAW LIFE SUPPORT AFTER CONSULTATION

I,_____, having been
designated by _____ to serve as health care surrogate
if this patient lacks capacity to make health care decisions and having
consulted with the patient's attending physician, agree that the following life
support be withheld or withdrawn:_____.

_____
Designee   Date

_____
Attending physician   Date

_____
Witness   Date

_____
Witness   Date

_____
Interpreter   Date

FORM 4.1.1.1
ALTERNATE REQUEST
BY SURROGATE, GUARDIAN, OR PROXY TO WITHHOLD
OR WITHDRAW LIFE-SUSTAINING PROCEDURES

Re: Patient _____ ,

I,_____, certify that I am authorized to direct that life-sustaining procedures be withheld or withdrawn on behalf of the above named patient by virtue of my relationship to the patient as (health care surrogate, court-appointed guardian, or legitimate proxy). I understand that the patient's attending physician and consulting physician have concluded that, in their medical opinion, the patient is terminally ill and lacks decision-making capacity.

I have had the opportunity to consult with the two physicians and all questions have been answered to my satisfaction. I am satisfied that the patient is in a terminal condition and lacks decision-making capacity with no reasonable probability of recovering capacity. Based on my reasonable belief that the patient would make this same decision had the patient been capable, I consent to and direct the withdrawal or withholding of life-sustaining procedures.

_____

Signature of surrogate or guardian or proxy   Date

_____

Attending physician   Date

_____

Witness   Date

_____

Witness   Date

_____

Interpreter   Date

FORM 4.2.1
HOSPITAL POLICY AND PROCEDURES—
WITHHOLDING AND WITHDRAWING LIFE-SUSTAINING
PROCEDURES FROM ADULT TERMINALLY ILL PATIENTS

POLICY

This hospital recognizes the right of competent adults to make an oral or written declaration directing the providing, withholding, or withdrawing of life-sustaining procedures or to designate another person to make treatment decisions.

Treatment decisions by a health care surrogate or proxy to withhold or withdraw life-sustaining procedures shall be based on the substituted judgment standard and his or her reasonable belief that the patient would make the same decision if the patient had decision-making capacity. Generally, decisions of the health care surrogate should be in accordance with the wishes, instructions, and conditions given in written or oral advance directives. Decisions by proxies should be supported by clear and convincing evidence that the decision would have been one the patient would have made capable of doing so.

I. PROCEDURES FOR A PATIENT WITH AN ADVANCE DIRECTIVE

A. Patient's Condition Should Be Assessed as Terminal

   Terminal condition means:

   1. A condition caused by injury, disease, or illness from which there is no reasonable probability of recovery and which, without treatment, can be expected to cause death; or

   2. A persistent vegetative state characterized by a permanent and irreversible condition of unconsciousness in which there is

      a. The absence of voluntary action or cognitive behavior of any kind; and

      b. An inability to communicate or interact purposefully with the environment.

B. Physician Documentation of Patient Condition

   1. *Determination of patient condition:* In determining whether the patient has a terminal condition or may recover capacity or whether a medical condition or limitation referred to in an advance directive exists, the patient's attending or treating

FORM 4.2.1 continued

physician and at least one other consulting physician must separately examine the patient. The findings of each examination must be documented in the patient's medical record on **Form 3.4.1** and signed by each examining physician before life-prolonging procedures may be withheld or withdrawn.

2. *Capacity of patient:* If the patient's capacity to make health care decisions or provide informed consent is in question, the attending physician and one other physician must separately evaluate the patient and conclude that the patient lacks capacity. The health care facility must enter both physicians' evaluations in the patient's clinical record, and the social services department or a patient representative must notify the health care surrogate in writing that his or her authority has commenced, if one has been designated.

3. *If the patient is pregnant:* If the patient is a female of childbearing age, the attending physician should document in the medical record whether the patient is pregnant or not. If she is pregnant, the medical management should progress on the merits of each case separately. If an advance directive expressly delegates authority to a surrogate to withhold or withdraw life-prolonging procedures from the pregnant patient prior to viability of the fetus, or if a surrogate or proxy has sought and received court approval, the advance directive may be followed. The attending physicians shall have access to separate members of the bioethics committee, an ad hoc committee, and/or hospital legal advisors for guidance and counsel on any case where withdrawing life support is an issue. Administration shall be notified.

C. Documentation or Discussion with Designated Decision Maker (Surrogate or Proxy) or Next-of-Kin

1. If the advance directive designates a surrogate to help make treatment decisions, that person must be contacted and consent by that person should be documented in the medical record, usually by signing **Form 4.1.1.1.**

2. If the advance directive does not designate a surrogate to execute the patient's wishes concerning life-prolonging procedures, a proxy must be appointed pursuant to the order of

FORM 4.2.1 continued

priority listed in section II.D.1 of this policy. Consent by that person should be documented in the medical record, usually by signing **Form 4.1.1.1**.

3. In cases where an interpreter assists, he or she should sign **Form 4.1.1.1** as interpreter.

4. If a surrogate or proxy cannot be found, the health care facility may proceed as directed by the patient on the advance directive.

5. The law does not require involvement of the next-of-kin when there is a valid advance directive. However, when the next-of-kin are present or can be reached by reasonable efforts within the time span of twenty-four hours, courtesy indicates that such efforts should be employed by the staff, not to secure their approval, but to keep them informed. The notification or an explanation of efforts to notify should be documented in the medical record. If the next-of-kin volunteer strong objections, hospital legal counsel should be consulted before treatment is withheld or withdrawn. (For further discussion see item F.)

D. The Attending Physician Initiates Orders Specifying Scope of Treatment

   1. After the determination is made to withhold or withdraw treatment, the attending physician should write orders specifying the scope of treatment to be withheld or withdrawn. Nutrition and hydration are not considered any different from any other artificial life-prolonging procedure. Palliative care (intended to give comfort and alleviate pain) will not be withheld or withdrawn.

   2. A do-no-resuscitate or no-code-blue order shall be written.

E. Transfer of Care of Patient

   A health care provider who refuses to comply with the declaration of a patient or the treatment decision of a surrogate shall make reasonable efforts to transfer the patient to another health care provider who will comply with the declaration or treatment decision. A health care provider is not required to commit any act which is contrary to his or her moral or ethical beliefs concerning life-prolonging procedures if the patient (1) is not in

Form 4.2.1 continued

an emergency condition and (2) has received written information upon admission informing the patient of policies of the health care provider regarding such moral or ethical beliefs.

A health care provider that is unwilling to carry out the wishes of the patient because of moral or ethical beliefs must within seven days either (1) transfer the patient to another health care provider and pay the costs for transporting the patient or (2) carry out the wishes of the patient or his or her surrogate if the patient has not been transferred, *unless* a court proceeding has been initiated.

F. Disagreement among the Parties

Family approval is not required, although it is encouraged. The advance directive should be honored if properly executed with participation of the health care surrogate or proxy. If there is any discord, significant others shall be informed that they should initiate court resolution of the matter. Neither the hospital nor the physician need initiate the litigation.

G. Procedural Digressions

Actual or intended digressions from this procedure shall be brought to the attention of administration through notification of the nursing office.

II. PROCEDURES FOR A PATIENT WITH NO ADVANCE DI-RECTIVE

A. The Patient's Condition Should Be Assessed as Being Terminal as Defined Above

B. Physician Documentation of Patient Condition

1. *Determination of patient condition:* In determining whether the patient has a terminal condition or may recover capacity, the patient's attending or treating physician and at least one other consulting physician must separately examine the patient. The findings of each examination must be documented in the patient's medical record on **Form 3.4.1** and signed by each examining physician before life-prolonging procedures may be withheld or withdrawn.

2. *Capacity of patient:* If the patient's capacity to make health care decisions or provide informed consent is in question, the attending physician and one other physician must separately

FORM 4.2.1 continued

evaluate the patient and conclude that the patient lacks capacity. The health care facility must enter both physicians' evaluations in the patient's clinical record. Use **Form 3.4.1**. A proxy should be appointed for the patient using the order of priority listed in section II.D outlined below.

3. *If the patient is pregnant:* If the patient is a female of childbearing age, the attending physician should document in the medical record whether the patient is pregnant or not. If she is pregnant, the medical management should progress on the merits of each case separately. The attending physicians shall have access to separate members of the bioethics committee, and ad hoc committee, and/or hospital legal advisors for guidance and counsel on any case where withdrawing life support is an issue. Administration shall be notified.

C. Request Patient to Sign an Advance Directive, if Appropriate

If a patient does not have an advance directive but wishes to sign one after admission, an advance directive will be supplied upon patient request. Pastoral care and/or social services will be available to consult with the patient. The patient will execute the advance directive, and a copy must be made a part of the patient's medical record.

D. Appointment of Patient's Proxy

1. *Priority of patient proxies:* Where there is no advance directive or health care surrogate, the decision to withhold or withdraw artificial life-prolonging procedures shall involve proxies in the following order of priority:

   a. The judicially appointed guardian who has been authorized to consent to medical treatment, if one has been previously appointed.

   b. The patient's spouse.

   c. An adult child of the patient, or if the patient has more than one adult child, a majority of the adult children who are reasonably available for consultation.

   d. A parent of the patient.

FORM 4.2.1 continued

e. An adult sibling of the patient, or if the patient has more than one sibling, a majority of the adult siblings who are reasonably available for consultation.

f. An adult relative of the patient who has exhibited special care and concern for the patient, who has maintained regular contact with the patient, and who is familiar with the patient's activities, health, and religious or moral beliefs.

g. A close friend of the patient. The close friend must present an affidavit to the health care facility or the attending or treating physician stating that he or she is a friend of the patient, is willing and able to become involved in the patient's health care, and has maintained such regular contact with the patient as to be familiar with the patient's activities, health, religious or moral beliefs, and wishes regarding medical care. See **Form 3.3.2.**

If no individual in a prior class is reasonably available, willing, and competent to act, persons in the next priority class may decide.

Documentation of attempts to contact a health care surrogate or proxy should be indicated in the patient's medical record.

2. Documentation of consent of patient's proxy:

   a. Any health care decision must be based on the proxy's informed consent and on the decision the proxy reasonably believes the patient would have made under the circumstances. Any decision to withhold or withdraw life-prolonging procedures must be supported by clear and convincing evidence that the decision would have been the one that the patient would have chosen had he or she been competent.

   b. If the proxy is not following the known intention of the patient, the hospital legal counsel should be consulted to determine whether judicial involvement is required.

3. **Form 4.1.1.1** shall be signed by the attending or treating physician, the proxy, and two witnesses.

4. In instances where **Form 4.1.1.1** will be signed by a proxy whose language is not English, the English copy will be signed

FORM 4.2.1 continued

after having been translated verbally by an interpreter. In all cases of participation by an interpreter, his or her signature shall appear on **Form 4.1.1.1** as witness/interpreter.

E. The Attending Physician Initiates Orders Specifying Scope of Treatment

1. After the determination is made to withhold or withdraw treatment, the attending physician should write orders specifying the scope of treatment to be withheld or withdrawn. Nutrition and hydration are not considered any different from any other artificial life-prolonging procedure. Palliative care (intended to give comfort and alleviate pain) will not be withheld or withdrawn.

2. A do-not-resuscitate or no-code-blue order shall be written.

F. Transfer of Care

A health care provider who refuses to comply with the treatment decision of a surrogate or proxy shall make reasonable efforts to transfer the patient to another health care provider who will comply with the treatment decision. A health care provider is not required to commit any act which is contrary to his or her moral or ethical beliefs concerning life-prolonging procedures if the patient (1) is not in an emergency condition and (2) has received written information upon admission informing the patient of policies of the health care provider regarding such moral or ethical beliefs.

A health care provider that is unwilling to carry out the wishes of the patient because of moral or ethical beliefs must within seven days either (1) transfer the patient to another health care provider and pay the costs for transporting the patient or (2) carry out the wishes of the patient or his or her surrogate if the patient has not been transferred, *unless* a court proceeding has been initiated.

G. Disagreement among the Parties

Family approval is not required, although it is encouraged. The advance directive should be honored if properly executed with participation of the health care surrogate or proxy. If there is any discord, significant others shall be informed that they should initiate court resolution of the matter. Neither the hospital nor the physician need initiate this litigation.

FORM 4.2.1 continued

H. Patients Without a Surrogate or Proxy

When necessary, the social services department will be contacted to expedite procedures for the appointment of a guardian for health care decision making.

I. Procedural Digressions

Actual or intended digressions from this procedure shall be brought to the attention of administration through notification of the nursing office.

FORM 4.2.2
HOSPITAL POLICY AND PROCEDURES—
WITHHOLDING AND WITHDRAWING LIFE-SUSTAINING
PROCEDURES FROM PEDIATRIC TERMINALLY ILL PATIENTS

POLICY

This hospital recognizes the right of a parent or guardian to make a written declaration instructing physician(s) to provide, withhold, or withdraw life-sustaining procedures or to make the treatment decisions for a minor patient in the event such patient is diagnosed as suffering from a terminal condition. A minor patient is one who has not attained the age of eighteen years and is not emancipated, that is, not married, not living independently and taking care of his or her own affairs, and not in the armed services.

I. PROCEDURES

A. The Patient's Condition Should be Assessed as Terminal

Terminal condition means:

1. A condition caused by injury, disease, or illness from which there is no reasonable probability of recovery and which, without treatment, can be expected to cause death; or

2. A persistent vegetative state characterized by a permanent and irreversible condition of unconsciousness in which there is

   a. The absence of voluntary action or cognitive behavior of any kind; and

   b. An inability to communicate or interact purposefully with the environment.

B. Physician Documentation of Patient Condition

1. *Determination of patient condition:* In determining whether the patient has a terminal condition, the patient's attending or treating physician and at least one other consulting physician must separately examine the patient. The findings of each examination must be documented in the patient's medical record on **Form 4.2.3** and signed by each examining physician before life-prolonging procedures may be withheld or withdrawn.

2. *If the patient is pregnant:* If the patient is a female of child-bearing age, the attending physician should document in the medical record whether the patient is pregnant or not. If she

FORM 4.2.2 continued

is pregnant, the medical management should progress on the merits of each case separately. The attending physicians shall have access to separate members of the bioethics committee, an ad hoc committee, and/or hospital legal advisors for guidance and counsel on any case where withdrawing life support is an issue. Administration shall be notified.

C. Appointment of Patient's Proxy

1. *Priority of patient proxies:* The decision to withhold or withdraw artificial life-prolonging procedures shall involve proxies in the following order of priority:

   a. The judicially appointed guardian who has been authorized to consent to medical treatment, if one has been previously appointed.

   b. A parent of the patient.

   If no individual in a prior class is reasonably available, willing, and competent to act, judicial proceedings to obtain a guardian will be initiated.

   Documentation of attempts to contact a health care surrogate or proxy should be indicated in the patient's medical record.

2. *Documentation of consent of patient's proxy:* Any health care decision must be based on the proxy's informed consent. The attending physician and the proxy must have at least two witnesses present at the consultation at which agreement is reached concerning withholding or withdrawing treatment.

3. **Form 4.2.4** shall be signed by the attending or treating physician, the proxy, and two witnesses.

4. In instances where **Form 4.2.4** will be signed by a proxy whose language is not English, the English copy will be signed after having been translated verbally by an interpreter. In all cases of participation by an interpreter, his or her signature shall appear on **Form 4.2.4** as witness/interpreter.

D. The Attending Physician Initiates Orders Specifying Scope of Treatment

1. After the determination is made to withhold or withdraw treatment, the attending physician should write orders specifying the scope of treatment to be withheld or withdrawn.

FORM 4.2.2 continued

Nutrition and hydration are not considered any different from any other artificial life-prolonging procedure. Palliative care (intended to give comfort and alleviate pain) will not be withheld or withdrawn.

2. A do-not-resuscitate or no-code-pink order shall be written.

E. Transfer of Care

A health care provider who refuses to comply with the treatment decision of a proxy shall make reasonable efforts to transfer the patient to another health care provider who will comply with the treatment decision. A health care provider is not required to commit any act which is contrary to his or her moral or ethical beliefs concerning life-prolonging procedures if the patient is not in an emergency condition.

A health care provider that is unwilling to carry out the wishes of the proxy because of moral or ethical beliefs must within seven days either (1) transfer the patient to another health care provider and pay the costs for transporting the patient or (2) carry out the wishes of the proxy if the patient has not been transferred, *unless* a court proceeding has been initiated.

F. Patients Without a Proxy

When necessary, the social services department will be contacted to expedite procedures for the appointment of a guardian for health care decision making.

G. Procedural Digressions

Actual or intended digressions from this procedure shall be brought to the attention of administration through notification of the nursing office.

FORM 4.2.3
CERTIFICATION OF PEDIATRIC TERMINAL CONDITION

Patient's name _____

We certify that the above patient has a terminal condition.

Terminal means (please check condition corresponding to patient diagnosis):

___1. A condition caused by injury, disease, or illness for which there is no reasonable probability of recovery and which, without treatment, can be expected to cause death; or

___2. A persistent vegetative state characterized by a permanent and irreversible condition of unconsciousness in which there is

    a. The absence of voluntary action or cognitive behavior of any kind, and

    b. An inability to communicate or interact purposefully with the environment.

___3. The patient has existed in such condition for at least a period of __months because of (check one):

    a. hypoxia-ischemia

    b. closed head injury

    c. other etiology (please list):_____

___4. There has been no improvement since this assessment for a period of at least ___months.

Documentation of Patient Assessment

We have examined the above named patient and have documented in the patient's medical record the objective criteria according to which we have made our assessments concerning the patient's terminal condition.

_____

Patient's attending physician   Date

_____

Patient's consulting physician   Date

FORM 4.2.3.1
ALTERNATE CLAUSE REGARDING DOCUMENTATION
OF ORAL CONSENT BY PROXY FOR WITHHOLDING
OR WITHDRAWING LIFE-SUSTAINING TREATMENT
FROM PEDIATRIC PATIENT

Form 4.2.4 shall be based on the proxy's informed consent, signed by the proxy, and also signed by the attending or treating physician and one witness. In those situations, however, where a proxy is unable or unwilling to affix his or her signature to the document but has given knowing and voluntary oral consent to the withholding or withdrawal of life-sustaining treatment after a consultation with and full explanation by the attending physician and without undue coercion or influence, the attending physician may dispense with the written document if in his or her medical judgment sufficient reasons exist for so doing and if the physician documents the reasons and the proxy's oral consent in the progress notes and the notes are signed by one witness who was present during the explanation to the proxy who attests to the reasons for the proxy's inability or unwillingness to sign the document and to the proxy's oral consent. This documentation shall have the same force and effect as if **Form 4.2.4** had been signed by the proxy.

FORM 4.2.3.2
OPTIONAL CLAUSE REGARDING
A MINOR'S PARTICIPATION IN DECISION MAKING

Where, in the medical judgment of the attending physician, an unemancipated minor is mature and capable of understanding an explanation of his or her physical condition and proposed procedures and also capable of making a knowing health care decision, such minor shall be allowed to participate in the decision to withhold or withdraw life-sustaining treatment, although the ultimate decision shall be made only by the proxy.

FORM 4.2.3.3
OPTIONAL CLAUSE TO ACCEPT
A MINOR'S DECISION TO WITHHOLD OR WITHDRAW
LIFE-SUSTAINING TREATMENT

Where, in the medical judgment of the attending physician, an unemancipated minor is mature and capable of understanding an explanation of his or her physical condition and proposed procedures and also capable of making a knowing health care decision, the minor's decision to withhold or withdraw life-sustaining treatment standing alone shall be accepted as valid and **Form 1.2.1** shall be signed by the minor, the attending physician, and one witness.

FORM 4.2.4
REQUEST BY PROXY TO WITHHOLD OR WITHDRAW LIFE-SUSTAINING PROCEDURES FROM PEDIATRIC PATIENT

Patient's name _____

I,_____, am the proxy for the above named patient. I understand that the patient's attending physician and consulting physician have concluded that, in their medical opinion, the patient is terminally ill.

I have had the opportunity to consult with the two physicians and all questions have been answered to my satisfaction. I am satisfied that the patient is in a terminal condition.

I request and consent to the withholding or withdrawal of life-sustaining procedures. It is my wish that the patient's suffering not be uselessly prolonged and to refuse burdensome life-sustaining procedures for the patient.

Proxy_____

_____   _____
Proxy's relationship   Date

_____   _____
Attending physician   Date

_____   _____
Witness   Date

_____   _____
Witness   Date

_____   _____
Interpreter   Date

FORM 5.1.1
CARDIOPULMONARY RESUSCITATION AND
DO-NOT-RESUSCITATE ORDERS: QUESTIONS AND ANSWERS

What is cardiopulmonary resuscitation?

Cardiopulmonary resuscitation (CPR) is an emergency procedure, such as mouth-to-mouth resuscitation, chest compression, or electric shock, which is routinely initiated to revive a patient whose heart or breathing has stopped. The purpose of CPR is to prevent sudden and unexpected death.

How successful is CPR?

It is not successful in many situations. The success rate of CPR can be judged by the fact that about two-thirds of patients do not survive CPR and approximately 15 percent of patients live until they are discharged from the hospital. In some cases, CPR is not indicated. In other cases, where it is used, it may be only partly successful and may result in severe damage to the brain or other organs.

Should patients discuss CPR with their physicians?

Yes. A patient should be actively involved in these discussions and should request them soon after being admitted to the hospital and while he or she is alert in order that the patient's diagnosis, prognosis, and suitability for CPR can be made clear, the risks and benefits of CPR can be explained, and the patient's wishes regarding CPR can be expressed to the physician.

Are patients entitled to refuse CPR?

All adults able to make an informed decision have the right under the laws of all states to accept or refuse medical procedures. This includes CPR. Instructions can be given orally or in a living will. Preferences about CPR can also be given to individuals appointed by a durable power of attorney or health care surrogate designation who will make proxy health care decisions for the patient who becomes unable to make these decisions. If a patient has made no living will, durable power of attorney, or health care surrogate designation and is not able to make a decision about CPR, another person, such as a guardian appointed by a court, a family member, or a close friend, can make the decision.

What is a do-not-resuscitate (DNR) order?

It is a physician's direction entered in the patient's medical record that no CPR is to be initiated. It is issued by the physician when the patient refuses CPR and consents to the order.

FORM 5.1.1 continued

If a patient consents to a DNR order, can the patient revoke it later?

If the patient has a change of heart or a change in medical condition, consent to the DNR order may be withdrawn by an oral or written statement made to the physician or nursing staff of the hospital.

If a DNR order is given, does this mean that a patient will not receive any other treatment?

The order only relates to cardiopulmonary (CPR) procedures. A patient will continue to be given comfort care and all other care, such as food, water, drugs, or antibiotics.

What happens if no DNR order is given by the doctor?

A trained staff member will initiate CPR measures for any patient who suffers cardiac or respiratory arrest.

What happens if the patient's physician does not agree with the patient's request for a DNR order?

If the patient's physician does not agree with the request, a consultation with another doctor or the chaplain or hospital ethics committee will be held, or the physician will arrange to transfer the care of the patient to another doctor.

FORM 5.1.2
REFUSAL OF
CARDIOPULMONARY RESUSCITATION AND RELEASE

I, _____,
refuse to allow the administration of any resuscitative procedure on me by my physician or the ABC Hospital.

I have received from my physician a full explanation about the seriousness of my condition and the risks to my life and health created by my refusal. I also understand the poor success ratio CPR has for adult patients as well as the damage it may cause to the brain and other organs.

I hereby release the hospital, any physicians connected with my care, and the nurses and employees of the hospital who have been or will be involved in my care from all liability and damages for injury to me or for my death for respecting my wishes and directions in this matter. This release includes a full release from all manner of causes of action or suits which I have or will have against the hospital or any physicians connected with my care by reason of respecting my wishes and directions.

I confirm that I have read and fully understand the above prior to my own signing.

_____   _____
Signature   Date

_____   _____
Attending physician   Date

_____   _____
Witness   Date

_____   _____
Witness   Date

_____   _____
Interpreter   Date

FORM 5.1.3
CONSENT TO NO CARDIOPULMONARY RESUSCITATION

I, _____,
hereby agree that cardiopulmonary resuscitation should not be administered
to me.

I have received from my physician a full explanation about the seriousness of
my condition and understand that resuscitation is not medically appropriate
for me and will not provide any medical benefit.

I confirm that I have read and fully understand the above prior to my own
signing.

_____   _____
Signature   Date

_____   _____
Witness   Date

_____   _____
Witness   Date

_____   _____
Interpreter   Date

FORM 5.1.4
DO-NOT-RESUSCITATE ORDER

Physician's name _____

Code Status:

____ NO Cardiopulmonary Resuscitation—All cardiopulmonary efforts are to be withheld.

____ LIMITED Cardiopulmonary Resuscitation—The following specific measures should be withheld:

    ____ ventilation by mask

    ____ endotracheal intubation

    ____ antiarrhythmics

    ____ mechanical ventilation

    ____ chest compression

    ____ intravenous vasoactive drugs

    ____ defibrillation/countershock

_____

Physician's signature   Date

FORM 5.2.1
HOSPITAL POLICY AND PROCEDURES—
DO-NOT-RESUSCITATE ORDER

POLICY

The purpose of this policy is to clarify the do-not-resuscitate order and the procedures to be followed in connection therewith. The ABC Hospital recognizes that the purpose of cardiopulmonary resuscitation (CPR) is the prevention of sudden, unexpected death. The order to resuscitate is a standing order of this hospital. In the event of cardiac or pulmonary arrest, CPR is to be initiated unless there is a specific do-not-resuscitate (DNR) order to the contrary. As with other medical procedures, however, there are clinical situations in which this procedure may be of uncertain medical value or medically futile and should not be implemented. There are also situations in which a patient may decide to forgo CPR. The ABC Hospital also recognizes the right to patient autonomy, that is, for a patient to participate in decisions affecting his or her life and to have his or her values and beliefs respected within the law. In any situation, the consent of the patient or surrogate or proxy to a DNR order is required.

DEFINITIONS

Cardiopulmonary resuscitation is a group of procedures employed to restore and maintain breathing and blood circulation in a patient who has suffered cardiac or pulmonary arrest.

A *do-not-resuscitate order* is a written medical order prepared by the attending physician that documents instructions by an adult patient, the patient's designated surrogate, or appointed proxy that in the event the patient suffers cardiac or pulmonary arrest, CPR is to be withheld.

Limited code, slow code, and *chemical code* are perfunctory procedures that fall short of full CPR.

DISCUSSIONS AND REFUSAL OF CPR

1. Attending physicians shall discuss with patients, or, if they lack decision-making capacity, with surrogates or proxies, the medical appropriateness of CPR. Physicians shall provide information about the patient's diagnosis and prognosis, the reasonably foreseeable risks and benefits of CPR in light of the patient's condition, and the consequences of a DNR order. Whether physicians have determined

FORM 5.2.1 continued

that CPR is appropriate or is futile, they shall explain in candid and detailed discussions their medical basis for its appropriateness or futility. Sufficient medical information shall be conveyed to allow an informed decision to be made.

2. A patient with decision-making capacity may, because of a chronic medical condition, wish to request no resuscitation even if CPR is appropriate. Have the patient complete a Refusal of CPR and Release (**Form 5.1.2**). If the patient is suffering from a terminal illness and already rejected CPR in a living will, this form need not be completed.

3. Two witnesses shall witness the physician's explanation. The witnesses shall sign **Form 5.1.2**.

4. The patient's refusal of CPR shall be honored by the attending physicians. Notify the nursing administration.

5. If the patient obviously lacks decision-making capacity, **Form 5.1.2** will not be signed and the attending physician will document this fact in the record. The evaluation by a second physician is not necessary.

6. If the lack of decision-making capacity is in question, the attending physician shall evaluate the patient's capacity and document the evaluation in the medical record. If the attending physician determines that the patient lacks capacity, the ABC Hospital shall have another physician, not employed by the hospital or associated with the attending physician, evaluate the patient's capacity. The second physician's evaluation, if in agreement with the attending physician's evaluation that the patient lacks capacity, shall also be documented in the medical record.

7. If a patient is obviously lacking in decision-making capacity, or if there is a question, and both physicians evaluate the patient as lacking capacity, the surrogate or proxy, after candid and detailed discussions with the attending physician as provided above, may wish to request no CPR even if CPR is appropriate. Have the surrogate or proxy complete **Form 1.3.4**.

8. Two witnesses shall witness the explanation and shall sign the form.

9. If the attending physician determines that the well-being of the patient would be adversely affected by a discussion of the patient's medical condition and the appropriateness or futility of CPR,

FORM 5.2.1 continued

discussion should be held with the surrogate or proxy concerning refusal of CPR. If the surrogate or proxy wishes to request no resuscitation, have him or her complete **Form 1.3.4.** Two witnesses shall also witness the explanation and shall sign the form.

IMPLEMENTATION OF DNR ORDER

10. If there is a refusal of CPR by a patient, surrogate, or proxy, the DNR order will be prepared by the attending physician and no other. It shall be in writing and shall be placed in the patient's chart. No oral or telephone orders shall be issued. In the chart there shall also be placed the diagnosis, prognosis, reasonably foreseeable risks and benefits of CPR, and the wishes or consent of the patient or representatives to the issuance of the DNR order. If issued, the DNR order only limits initiation of cardiopulmonary resuscitation. It is compatible with maximal therapeutic care or supportive care.

PATIENT'S REFUSAL TO CONSENT TO DNR ORDER

11. The DNR order shall not be written if the patient, surrogate, or proxy is not in agreement as to the inappropriateness of the application of CPR and does not consent to a DNR order.

12. A physician has no moral obligation to make CPR available to a patient when, in the physician's judgment, CPR is clearly futile. The physician shall be readily available, openly candid, and detailed in explaining to the patient, surrogate, or proxy the physician's medical basis for the futility of CPR. However, in the event of a disagreement with the physician concerning the administration of CPR, a second opinion or consultation with facilitators such as the chaplain or ethics committee may be desirable. If such consultation fails to resolve the question, the patient, surrogate, or proxy shall be informed of arrangements to transfer the patient to another physician. If no physician is willing to accept the case under the conditions stipulated by the patient, surrogate, or proxy, hospital counsel will be notified to consider relief through a court proceeding.

REVOCATION

13. If a DNR order has been issued based on consent, whether because of changed conditions, such as an improvement in the patient's

FORM 5.2.1 continued

clinical condition, an error in the original diagnosis, or the development of a new therapy, or otherwise, a patient, surrogate, or proxy may later at any time revoke the DNR order by oral or written declaration to the physician or nursing staff. Upon notification of the revocation, the physician shall immediately document such revocation in the patient's chart, cancel the DNR order, and notify the nursing staff.

14. If, because of changed conditions, the physician believes that the DNR order should be revoked, the physician should explain carefully the reasons to the patient with decision-making capacity or to the proxy or surrogate if the patient lacks such capacity.

15. In the event of a disagreement with the physician concerning the revocation by the patient, surrogate, or proxy or the revocation recommended by the physician, a second opinion or consultation with facilitators such as the chaplain or ethics committee may be desirable. If such consultation fails to resolve the question, the patient's, proxy's, or surrogate's revocation shall stand or the physician-proposed revocation shall be rejected.

16. A physician has no moral obligation to make CPR available to a patient when, in the physician's judgment, CPR is clearly futile. The physician has no moral obligation to withhold CPR when the physician believes that doing so will harm the patient. If such judgments are made, the case will be governed by section 12 of this policy.

LIMITED CODE, SLOW CODE, AND CHEMICAL CODE

17. Limited code, slow code, and chemical code are not considered standard CPR.

18. Perfunctory CPR is unnecessary and leads to misunderstanding among nursing staff, physician, and proxies or surrogates. Physicians have an obligation to explain that procedures short of full CPR are unlikely to be successful.

19. DNR orders do not preclude treatment to alleviate pain or other medical conditions such as respiratory distress.

FORM 5.2.1 continued

TEMPORARY SUSPENSION OF DNR ORDERS

20. Patients with terminal conditions may have DNR orders in place to avoid CPR when the natural course of their disease reaches the final stages.

21. Instances may arise when it is appropriate to temporarily suspend the DNR order. The physician should carefully explain to the patient, proxy, or surrogate the reason for suspension, the duration, and objectives.

22. Examples include (but are not limited to) a temporary medical problem which is easily correctable; palliative surgery for a pathologic fracture; and surgery for an unrelated condition (transurethral prostatic resection [TURP] in a cancer patient).

FORM 5.2.1.1
OPTIONAL CLAUSE PERMITTING DOCUMENTATION
OF ORAL REFUSAL OF CPR BY SURROGATE OR PROXY

If any situation arises in which a surrogate or proxy is unable or unwilling to affix his or her signature to **Form 1.3.4** but has given knowing and voluntary refusal of resuscitative treatment after a consultation with and full explanation by the attending physician and without undue coercion or influence, the attending physician may dispense with the written document if in his or her medical judgment sufficient reasons exist for so doing and if the physician documents the reasons and the surrogate or proxy's oral refusal in the progress notes and the notes are signed by one witness who was present during the explanation to the surrogate or proxy who attests to the reasons for the surrogate's or proxy's inability or unwillingness to sign the document and to the surrogate's or proxy's oral refusal. This documentation shall have the same force and effect as if **Form 1.3.4** had been signed by the surrogate or proxy.

FORM 5.2.1.2
DO-NOT-RESUSCITATE PROGRESS NOTES

Re: Patient _____

Notes on explanation to patient regarding do-not-resuscitate order:

   a. Discussion with patient about seriousness of medical condition and risks and medical inappropriateness of CPR.

   b. Patient's understanding and agreement.

   c. Registered nurse witnessed discussion.

   d. Assessment of patient's decision-making capacity and any adverse effects from a disclosure of patient's condition.

   e. Patient signed consent for no CPR (**Form 5.1.2**). Form signed by registered nurse.

_____

Physician   Date

_____

Registered nurse   Date

FORM 5.2.1.3
OPTIONAL CLAUSE
TO EXPEDITE GUARDIANSHIP PROCEEDINGS

In the event a patient lacks decision-making capacity and has not designated a surrogate and it appears that no individuals authorized to act as legitimate proxies for the patient will or can be found, the social services department will be contacted immediately to expedite procedures for the appointment of a guardian authorized to make health care decisions.

FORM 5.2.2
ALTERNATE HOSPITAL POLICY AND
PROCEDURES—DO-NOT-RESUSCITATE ORDER

POLICY

The purpose of this policy is to clarify the actions to be taken in the event a patient suffers cardiac or pulmonary arrest.

PROCEDURES

Cardiopulmonary Procedures

1. When a patient suffers cardiac or pulmonary arrest, aggressive cardiopulmonary resuscitation (CPR) procedures following the guidelines on advanced cardiac life support and the American Heart Association will be initiated by a trained staff member except when a do-not-resuscitate (DNR) order has been placed in the patient's medical record.

2. After such procedures have been initiated, they shall be discontinued only when a written specific do-not-resuscitate order has been issued by the attending physician.

3. Such procedures shall not be initiated if a do-not-resuscitate order in writing has been entered in the patient's medical record by the attending physician. The DNR order will be followed by every staff member.

Entry of Do-Not-Resuscitate Order

4. A do-not-resuscitate order may be entered if:

   a. In the attending physician's judgment, arrived at after consultation with the primary service providers, the patient has no reasonable hope of survival and CPR is clearly futile. Examples of a futile intervention include, but are not limited to, (1) one with no pathophysiologic rationale; (2) one that has already failed; (3) one that will not achieve the goals of care; or (4) one that would occur after maximal treatment has failed. The physician is not morally obligated to comply with a patient's, surrogate's, or proxy's request or direction for an intervention or offer the intervention when the physician considers it futile. The physician shall document in the progress notes in detail the

FORM 5.2.2 continued

medical basis for futility of the intervention and shall give to the patient, surrogate, or proxy an explanation of it sufficient to allow him or her to understand the medical basis for the futility of the intervention. The patient, surrogate, or proxy shall be informed of the DNR order but not offered the choice of the DNR order.

b. A patient with decision-making capacity refuses CPR.

c. In cases where the patient lacks such capacity, the patient's surrogate or proxy refuses CPR.

Consultation

5. If a patient, surrogate, or proxy requests no CPR:

a. The attending physician shall explore the reason for the request and document the discussion in the medical record by means of a progress note.

b. Consultation with another physician is to be held if the patient has decision-making capacity. The other physician shall also document in the medical record by means of a progress note the discussion and his or her opinion that the request is or is not warranted.

c. Consultation with another physician is to be held if the patient lacks decision-making capacity and has an advance directive. The other physician shall document in the medical record whether the request is or is not in line with the advance directive.

d. Consultation with another physician is to be held where the patient lacks decision-making capacity and has made no advance directive and where the request is made by a proxy. The other physician shall document in the medical record his or her opinion whether the request is or is not warranted.

e. Consultation with facilitators such as the chaplain or ethics committee is desirable if (1) there is no agreement between the attending physician and the second physician or (2) if there is no agreement between the physician(s) and the patient, surrogate, or proxy.

FORM 5.3.1
PREHOSPITAL DO-NOT-RESUSCITATE ORDER

Patient's name_____

Effective date: _____

Attending Physicians Order

I, _____, a physician
licensed under the laws of this state, state that I am the attending physician
of the above named patient. I have documented in the patient's medical
record that: (must check 1 or 2)

___1. The patient is capable of making an informed decision and consent
about providing, withholding, or withdrawing a specific medical
treatment or course of treatment. (Signature of patient is required
in section A below.)

___2. The patient is incapable of making an informed decision and
consent about providing, withholding, or withdrawing a specific
medical treatment because the patient is unable to understand the
nature, extent, or probable consequences of the proposed medical
decision or to make a rational evaluation of the risks and benefits of
alternatives to that decision. I have made this determination after
consultation with another physician licensed under the laws of this
state.

If 2 is checked above, either 1, 2, or 3 must be checked:

___1. The patient has executed a written advance directive which directs
that life-sustaining procedures be withheld or withdrawn. (Signature of surrogate, guardian, or proxy is required in section B and a
copy of the advance directive must be attached.)

___2. The patient has executed a written advance directive which appoints
a health care surrogate to make health care decisions on behalf of
the patient and provides that surrogate with authority to direct that
life-prolonging procedures be withheld or withdrawn. (Signature of
the appointed surrogate is required in section B and a copy of the
advance directive must be attached.)

___3. The patient has not executed an advance directive. (Signature of
guardian, if one has been appointed, or proxy is required in section
B.)

FORM 5.3.1 continued

Based on the informed directive, decision, and consent in section A or B, I hereby direct any and all emergency medical services personnel, commencing on the effective date noted above, to withhold cardiopulmonary resuscitation from the patient in the event of the patient's cardiac or respiratory arrest. I further direct such personnel to provide to the patient other medical interventions, such as intravenous fluids, oxygen, or other therapies, deemed necessary to provide comfort care or to alleviate pain.

_____

Attending physician's printed name

_____

Attending physician's signature

_____

Phone

_____

Physician's medical license number

This DNR form has been properly completed.

_____

Signature of patient or health care surrogate or court-appointed guardian or proxy

FORM 5.3.1 continued

Section A
Patient's Signature

I, the undersigned, hereby direct that in the event of my cardiac or respiratory arrest efforts at cardiopulmonary resuscitation not be initiated. I understand that I may revoke these directions at any time by physical cancellation or destruction of this form; or by orally expressing a desire to be resuscitated to EMS personnel; or by means of a subsequently executed advance directive that is materially different from this order. I also understand that if EMS personnel have any doubts about the applicability or validity of this order, they will begin cardiopulmonary resuscitation.

_____

Patient's printed name

_____

Patient's signature   Date

_____

Witness's printed name

_____

Witness's signature   Date

_____

Witness's printed name

_____

Witness's signature   Date

FORM 5.3.1 continued

Section B
Signature of Health Care Surrogate,
Court-Appointed Guardian, or Proxy

I, the undersigned, hereby certify that I am authorized to provide consent on the patient's behalf by virtue of my relationship to the patient as: _____

In that capacity, and based upon my reasonable belief that the patient would make this same decision under these circumstances had the patient been capable, I hereby direct that in the event of the patient's cardiac or respiratory arrest, efforts at cardiopulmonary resuscitation not be initiated. I understand that I may revoke these directions at any time by physical cancellation or destruction of this form; or by orally expressing a desire that the patient be resuscitated to EMS personnel; or by means of a subsequently executed advance directive that is materially different from this order. I also understand that if EMS personnel have any doubts about the applicability or validity of this order, they will begin cardiopulmonary resuscitation of the patient.

_____

Printed name of health care surrogate
or court-appointed guardian or proxy

_____

Signature of health care surrogate   Date
or court-appointed guardian or proxy

_____

Witness's printed name

_____

Witness's signature   Date

_____

Witness's printed name

_____

Witness's signature   Date

FORM 6.1.1
YOUR RIGHTS TO MAKE
HEALTH CARE DECISIONS AND ADVANCE DIRECTIVES

According to this state's law, every adult has the fundamental right to control decisions about his or her medical treatment. Further, the rights and intentions of a person may be respected even after he or she is no longer able to make decisions or to communicate those decisions. You can find this law in the statutes of this state, Secs._____.

Each person has the right to decide whether to accept or reject treatment, including decisions involving the withholding or withdrawing of life-sustaining procedures and the artificial provision of food and water under certain conditions. The law recognizes that an adult while able to make medical treatment decisions may designate another person to substitute as decision maker or surrogate for when the adult has become incapacitated. Any limit to the power of the substitute or surrogate should be clearly expressed.

This right applies where the adult expressed his or her desires in a written advance directive, such as a living will; in oral declarations established by clear and convincing evidence; or by the written designation of a substitute decision maker such as a durable power of attorney, health care surrogate, court-appointed guardian, or other health care decision maker.

The ABC Hospital recognizes the individual's right to make decisions concerning medical care, including the right to accept or refuse medical or surgical treatment, the right to accept or refuse life-sustaining procedures, and the right to formulate advance directives. An *advance directive* as referred to in this policy is defined as a living will, a durable power of attorney, or a designation of a health care surrogate.

In accordance with the Omnibus Reconciliation Act of 1991 and this state's laws, the ABC Hospital ascertains at the time of admission if the individual has executed an advance directive and notes this information in the patient's records.

Additionally , the ABC Hospital recognizes its responsibility to provide our patients with information regarding advance directives or living wills.

The provision of quality health care at the ABC Hospital is not based on whether or not the individual has executed an advance directive.

If you should require more information on advance directives, please contact our chaplain or our social services department.

FORM 6.1.2
ADVANCE DIRECTIVES BROCHURE

Advance directives are oral or written statements made in advance of serious illness. Through advance directives you can ensure that your wishes and rights will be carried out even if you are unconscious or cannot make your decisions known. There are three kinds of documents, and each has a different purpose. They offer different kinds of protection. One or more may be completed by you. The law does not prevent an individual from completing some or all of these documents for maximum protection in future medical situations. Advance directives were invented to allow us to plan ahead and to have a voice in decisions about our future medical treatment even when we are too sick to speak for ourselves. If we don't make this choice through an advance directive, someone else will choose for us.

The most well-known form of advance directive is called a *living will*. This document records and states your intentions and choices regarding health care and gives instructions about medical treatment. It is a document in which you can decide the kind of life-sustaining care you want. The living will, unlike the ordinary will, does not require that a person be dead before it is effective. But it is important to note what is legally necessary before it becomes effective. It cannot be given effect and your wishes cannot be carried out unless you are terminally ill. A living will also becomes effective only if the individual becomes incompetent.

To make the living will legal, it is not necessary that it be notarized. The law requires only that it be signed by you on the line above the word "Signature" and dated. It should be signed in the presence of two people, preferably people who know you well. At least one of the witnesses must be someone who is not your spouse or blood relative. The person designated as surrogate must not be a witness. If you cannot sign the living will because of physical disability, one of the witnesses can sign it for you at your request and in your presence. They should sign as witnesses in the spaces provided and fill in the date.

A *health care surrogate designation* allows you to appoint another person to make health care decisions and to provide informed consent. This is the second kind of advance directive. Again as in the living will, the condition is that you be incompetent. Note the language "in the event that I have been determined to be incapacitated to provide informed consent" for certain procedures. The health care surrogate can provide consent for treatment and also have your wishes about life-prolonging procedures carried out. If you have no living will, the surrogate can decide to withhold or withdraw

FORM 6.1.2 continued

life-sustaining procedures unless you have limited your surrogate's authority in this respect. This document has a distinct advantage over the living will since it allows a person you trust to make decisions for you whenever you cannot make your own in nonterminal situations. The health care surrogate can act not only when you have a terminal condition or are permanently vegetative but also at any other time when you may be seriously ill and not able to make your own decisions—as when you have been in a car accident, for example.

If you have appointed a person as surrogate under a living will, to avoid confusion, the same person should be appointed by a health care surrogate designation. You are also able to designate a backup surrogate. The alternate surrogate will take over if the first person you name is unwilling, unable, or unavailable to act for you.

To make this document legal, the law does not require notarization. But it requires that after you complete the form with the names of your surrogates, you sign the form at the end and date it. The form should be signed in the presence of two adult witnesses who also sign the form. If you cannot physically sign the form, one of the witnesses can sign it for you in your presence. The individuals you appoint as surrogates cannot act as witnesses. At least one of the witnesses must not be your spouse or a blood relative.

There is a third kind of advance directive also recognized by the law: a *durable power of attorney*. All states recognize a durable power of attorney. It permits you to appoint another person as attorney-in-fact with authority to manage your personal and business affairs—for example, collect rents, start or defend lawsuits, sign checks, and hire employees. You can include giving medical decision-making authority also, or you can make a durable power of attorney for health care which gives authority to the agent to arrange for your medical, therapeutic, and surgical procedures. Like the other forms of advance directives, it becomes effective if you become incapable of making medical decisions. Like the health care surrogate designation, it is effective in nonterminal situations. It must be signed by you and witnessed by two people, as with the living will and health care surrogate designation.

For further information about these advance directives, please contact our chaplain or our social services department.

FORM 6.1.3
INFORMATION FOR PHYSICIAN'S PATIENTS

The law of this state permits all of my patients to accept or refuse medical treatment and to make advance directives to give me instructions about their future medical care if they are not capable of communicating with me because of their condition. Advance directives include a living will—which gives directions if the patient has a terminal condition; a health care surrogate designation—which designates a person who will make health care decisions if a patient is not able to do so; or a durable power of attorney—which appoints another person to make decisions for the patient, including health care decisions.

OPTIONAL CLAUSES

- Patients who have made advance directives are requested to provide my office with a copy and I will honor them as well as any treatment decisions made by a health care surrogate or attorney-in-fact designated by my patients.

- Patients who have made advance directives are requested to provide my office with a copy. However, since my beliefs prevent me from complying with any directives which will produce the death of a patient, I will make every reasonable effort to transfer patients with such directives to another physician who will comply with their directives or the treatment decisions of a health care surrogate or attorney-in-fact designated by them.

FORM 6.1.4
ADVANCE DIRECTIVE FOLLOW-UP CHECKLIST

Hospital Representative:

Name _____

Title _____

(check or delete items where appropriate)

____ Patient states ___(did) ___(did not) receive written information from this hospital regarding his or her rights to accept or refuse medical or surgical treatment and to make advance directives.

PATIENT WITH ADVANCE DIRECTIVE

____ Patient made an advance directive prior to admission:
___LW   ___HCSD   ___DPAHC*

____ Patient ___(did) ___(did not) provide a copy of the advance directive to the hospital.

____ Patient ___(does) ___(does not) wish to change or revoke it.

PATIENT WITH NO ADVANCE DIRECTIVE

____ Patient made no advance directive prior to admission.

____ Patient was given the opportunity to ask questions about his or her rights concerning medical treatment and advance directives.

____ Patient was offered forms of advance directives and told how to complete them.

____ Patient ___(did) ___(did not) complete an advance directive. If patient completed one, patient ___(did) ___(did not) provide the hospital representative with a copy. ___LW   ___HCSD   ___DPAHC*

____ Patient designated the following health care surrogate to make medical decisions in the event the patient was physically or mentally unable to do so:

Name _____

Address_____Phone _____

_____

Hospital Representative   Date

This checklist is to be placed in the patient's medical record.

* LW = Living will; HCSD = Health care surrogate designation; DPAHC = Durable power of attorney for health care

FORM 6.2.1
HOSPITAL POLICY AND PROCEDURES—
IMPLEMENTATION OF PATIENTS' RIGHTS REGARDING
MEDICAL TREATMENT AND ADVANCE DIRECTIVES

POLICY

The ABC Hospital has heretofore established a policy which recognizes patient autonomy and the rights of patients with decision-making capacity, or of their proxies or surrogates if they lack such capacity, to accept or refuse all medical treatment. Its policy entitled Refusal of Treatment by Patients with Decision-Making Capacity and by Patients Without Decision-Making Capacity (**Form 1.3.1**) is incorporated herein by reference. This hospital also has an established policy entitled Patients with Advance Directives (**Form 3.3.1**), incorporated herein by reference, which recognizes an adult's right to formulate an advance directive.

An advance directive means a witnessed written document or oral statement in which instructions are given by a principal or in which the principal's desires are expressed concerning any aspect of the principal's health care.

An *advance directive* as referred to in this policy is defined as a living will, a durable power of attorney, or a health care surrogate designation.

In accordance with the Omnibus Reconciliation Act of 1991 and laws of this state, the ABC Hospital ascertains at the time of admission if the individual has executed an advance directive and notes this information in the patient's records.

Additionally , the ABC Hospital recognizes its responsibility to provide our patients with information regarding advance directives or living wills. The ABC Hospital is also committed to ensuring compliance with the requirements of this state's law respecting advance directives.

The provision of quality health care at the ABC Hospital is not based on whether or not the individual has executed an advance directive.

Furthermore, it is the policy of the ABC Hospital to provide for education of our staff and the local community on the issues concerning advance directives.

PROCEDURES

1. At the time of admitting adult in-patients into the ABC Hospital, they will be given information describing their rights under the laws

FORM 6.2.1 continued

of this state to accept or refuse medical treatment and to formulate advance directives and describing this hospital's policy to implement these rights.

Optional Clauses

- The information will be contained in Your Rights to Make Health Care Decisions and Advance Directives (**Form 6.1.1**).
- The information will be contained in the Advance Directives Brochure (**Form 6.1.2**).

2. At the time of admission, the hospital designee ascertains and documents into the individual's medical record as to whether or not the individual has executed an advance directive.

3. When an advance directive has been made, the procedures prescribed in this hospital's policy for reviewing and documenting it, which are contained in Patients with Advance Directives (**Form 3.3.1**), will be followed. The form is incorporated here by reference.

4. When an individual has no advance directive and requests information regarding advance directives or living wills, provisions are made for additional education materials by designated staff members, for example, social services, patient representatives, patient education, and so on. This may include related videos and appropriate forms to initiate advance directives. Nondesignated staff members should refer individuals requesting information to the appropriate designated staff members. Staff members (both designated and nondesignated) should encourage individuals to learn more about advance directives; however, they should refrain from answering specific questions or giving opinions on the law concerning advance directives. When specific questions on the law concerning advance directives are directed to staff members, the individual should be instructed to consult with his or her personal attorney.

5. The attending physician, any consulting physician, and other professional personnel shall provide the patient and/or his or her designee with information sufficient to enable him or her to make informed health care decisions for the patient. The designee's right to consultation, information, and cooperation is equal to that of the patient.

FORM 6.2.1 continued

6. With respect to the withholding or withdrawing of life-sustaining procedures: (1) when an advance directive has been made, the patient's condition should be assessed and documented and discussions with designated decision makers should be documented in accordance with the procedures prescribed in section I of this hospital's policy entitled Withholding and Withdrawing Life-Sustaining Procedures from Adult Terminally Ill Patients (**Form 4.2.1**); (2) when no advance directive has been made in the case of an adult patient, the patient's condition, including pregnancy, and capacity should be assessed and documented and a proxy appointed in accordance with the procedures prescribed in section II of said policy. This policy is incorporated herein by reference.

7. The attending physician who refuses to comply with the declaration of a qualified patient or the treatment decision of a person designated to make the decision by the declarant in his or her declaration shall make a reasonable effort to transfer the patient to another physician.

8. The hospital, physician, or other person who acts under the direction of a physician is not subject to criminal prosecution or civil liability, and will not be deemed to have engaged in unprofessional conduct, as a result of complying with the provisions of the individual's advance directive, or as a result of complying with the decision of a qualified patient's designee.

9. A person who acts in accordance with a qualified person's declaration is not subject to criminal prosecution or civil liability for such action.

10. This policy and specific policies relative to the implementation of patient rights shall be furnished to the individual and/or designee upon request and shall be maintained in a reference manual in each of the patient care units and in the admitting office.

Legal Citations

1. Brophy v. New England Mt. Sinai Hospital, Inc., 398 Mass. 417, 497 N.E.2d 626 (Supreme Judicial Court of Massachusetts, 1986).

2. Cruzan v. Director, Missouri Department of Health, 497 U.S. 261, 111 L.Ed.2d 224, 110 S.Ct. 841 (1990); Cruzan v. Harmon, 760 S.W. 2d 408 (Missouri Supreme Court, 1988).

3. Rasmussen v. Fleming, 741 P.2d 674 (Arizona Supreme Court, 1987); Bouvia v. Superior Court, 179 Cal. App. 3rd 1127, 225 Cal. Rptr. 297 (California Court of Appeal, 2d Appellate District, Division Two, 1986), *rev. den.* June 5, 1986; Bartling v. Superior Court of California, 163 Cal. App. 3rd 186, 209 Cal. Rptr. 220 (California Court of Appeal, 1984); Barber v. Superior Court of California, 174 Cal. App. 3rd 1006, 195 Cal. Rptr. 484 (California Court of Appeal, 2d District, 1983); John F. Kennedy Memorial Hospital, Inc. v. The Honorable Donald H. Bludworth, 452 So.2d 921 (Florida Supreme Court, 1984); In re Quinlan, 70 N.J. 10, 355 A.2d 647, *cert. den. sub. nom.*; Garger v. New Jersey, 429 U.S. 922 (1976); New Mexico *ex. rel.* Smith v. Fort, No. 14, 768 (New Mexico Supreme Court, 1983); Delio v. Westchester County Medical Center, 129 A.D.2d 1, 516 N.Y.S.2d 677 (New York Supreme Court, Appellate Division, 2d Department, 1987); Eichner v. Dillon, 73 A.D.2d 431, 426 N.Y.S.2d 517, *rev. sub. nom.* In re Storar, 52 N.Y. 2d 363, 420 N.E.2d 64, 438 N.Y.S.2d 266 (New York Court of Appeals), *cert. den.* 454 U.S. 858 (1981); Leach v. Shapiro, 13 Ohio App. 3rd 393, 469 N.E.2d 1047 (Ohio Court of Appeals for Summit County, 1984).

4. Natanson v. Kline, 186 Kan. 393, 406–407, 350 P. 2d 1093, 1104 (Kansas Supreme Court, 1960).

5. Union Pacific Railway Co. v. Botsford, 141 U.S. 250, 251 (1851).

6. Pratt v. Davis, 188 Ill. App. 161, 166, *aff'd* 224 Ill. 30, 79 N.E. 562 (Illinois Supreme Court, 1906).

7. Schloendorff v. Society of New York Hospital, 211 N.Y. 125, 129–130, 105 N.E. 92, 93 (New York Court of Appeals, 1914).

8. Matter of Claire Conroy, 98 N.J. 321, 486 A.2d 1209 (New Jersey Supreme Court, 1985); Cobbs v. Grant, 8 Cal. 3rd 229, 104 Cal. Rptr. 505, 502 P.2d 1 (California Supreme Court, 1972); Erickson v. Delgard, 44 Misc.2d 27, 252 N.Y.S.2d 705 (New York Supreme Court, 1962); Palm Springs General Hospital, Inc. v. Martinez, Civil No. 71-12687 (Florida, Dade County Circuit Court, July 2, 1971).

9. 381 U.S. 479 (1965).

10. 410 U.S. 113 (1973).

11. In re Quinlan, see *supra*, note 3.

12. Superintendent of Belchertown State School v. Saikewicz, 373 Mass. 728, 370 N.E.2d 417 (Supreme Judicial Court of Massachusetts, 1977); Satz v. Perlmutter, 362 So.2d 160, *aff'd* 379 So.2d 359 (Florida Supreme Court, 1980).

13. See *supra*, note 1, 497 N.E.2d at 634.

14. See *supra*, note 2.

15. 32 Ill. 2d 361, 205 N.E.2d 435 (Illinois Supreme Court, 1965).

16. People v. Pierson, 176 N.Y. 201, 68 N.E. 243 (New York Court of Appeals, 1903).

17. 58 N.J. 576, 279 A.2d 670 (New Jersey Supreme Court, 1971).

18. Matter of Claire Conroy, see *supra*, note 8; Bartling v. Superior Court, see *supra*, note 3.

19. McConnell v. Beverly Enterprises-Connecticut, Inc., 209 Conn. 692, 553 A.2d 596 (Connecticut Supreme Court, 1989).

20. People v. Pierson, see *supra*, note 16.

21. Application of the President and Directors of Georgetown College, 331 F.2d 1000 (District of Columbia Circuit Court), *cert. den.* 377 U.S. 978 (1964).

22. Wons v. Public Health Trust, 541 So.2d 96 (Florida Supreme Court, 1989); In re Osborne, 294 A.2d 372 (District of Columbia Court of Appeals, 1972).

23. Matter of Claire Conroy, see *supra*, note 8, 486 A.2d at 1225.

24. In re Quinlan, see *supra*, note 3, 355 A.2d at 664.

25. In re Storar, see *supra*, note 3.

26. Cruzan v. Harmon, see *supra*, note 2.

27. Cruzan v. Director, Missouri Department of Health, see *supra*, note 2.

28. Cruzan v. Director, Missouri Department of Health, see *supra*, note 2; Bartling v. Superior Court, see *supra*, note 3; Bouvia v. Superior Court, see *supra*, note 3.

29. Matter of Claire Conroy, see *supra*, note 8; Brophy v. New England Mt. Sinai Hospital, Inc., see *supra*, note 1; In re Guardianship of Estelle M. Browning, 543 So.2d 258, *aff'd* 568 So.2d (Florida Supreme Court, 1990).

30. Satz v. Perlmutter, see *supra*, note 12.

31. Brophy v. New England Mt. Sinai Hospital, Inc., see *supra*, note 1, 497 N.E.2d at 641.

32. In re Jobes, 108 N.J. 394, 529 A.2d 434 (New Jersey Supreme Court, 1987); Matter of Claire Conroy, see *supra*, note 8; Bouvia v. Superior Court, see *supra*, note 3; In re Peter, 108 N.J. 365, 529 A.D.2d 419 (New Jersey Supreme Court, 1987); Rasmussen v. Fleming, see *supra*, note 3; Barber v. Superior Court of California, see *supra*, note 3; Delio v. Westchester County Medical Center, see *supra*, note 3; Corbett v. D'Allessandro, 487 So.2d 368, *rev. den.* 492 So.2d 1331 (Florida Supreme Court, 1981).

33. See *supra*, note 2.

34. Brophy v. New England Mt. Sinai Hospital, Inc., see *supra*, note 1, 497 N.E.2d at 632.

35. In re Jobes, see *supra*, note 32.

36. In re Requena, 213 N.J. Super. 475, 517 A.2d 886, *aff'd* 213 N.J. Super. 443, 517 A.2d 869 (New Jersey Supreme Court, Appellate Division, 1986).

37. See *supra*, note 3, 209 Cal. Rptr. at 225.

38. Gray v. Romeo, 697 F. Supp. 580 (U.S. District Court, District Rhode Island, 1988).

39. In re Requena, see *supra*, note 36.

40. Hathaway v. Worcester City Hospital, 475 F.2d 701 (U.S. Court of Appeals, First Circuit, 1973).

41. See *supra*, note 12, 370 N.E.2d at 434.

42. In re Spring, 380 Mass. 629, 405 N.E. 115 (Supreme Judicial Court of Massachusetts, 1980).

43. In re Jobes, see *supra*, note 32, 529 A.2d at 451.

44. In re Quinlan, see *supra*, note 3, 355 A.2d at 669.

45. Florida Statutes, sec. 765.105.

46. For example, Florida Statutes, sec. 765.101 (17)(a) and (b).

47. Florida Statutes, sec. 765.03 (3) (1987, but amended in 1990).

48. Florida Statutes, sec. 765.075 (1990); Oklahoma Statutes, tit. 63, secs. 3080.1–3080.5 (amended in 1990 to permit refusal of artificial feeding via a living will).

49. Florida Statutes, sec. 765.075 (b)(2) (repealed in 1992).

50. Cruzan v. Harmon, see *supra*, note 2.

51. Cruzan v. Director, Missouri Department of Health, see *supra*, note 2.

52. In re Storar, see *supra*, note 3.

53. Cruzan v. Harmon, see *supra*, note 2.

54. Meyer v. Nebraska, 262 U.S. 390 (1923); Pierce v. Society of Sisters, 268 U.S. 501 (1927); In re Farrell, 108 N.J. 335, 529 A.2d 404 (New Jersey Supreme Court, 1987).

55. Parham, Commissioner, Department of Human Resources of Georgia v. J. R., 442 U.S. 585 (1925).

56. Matter of Claire Conroy, see *supra*, note 8.

57. Superintendent of Belchertown State School v. Saikewicz, see *supra*, note 12.

58. In re Quinlan, see *supra*, note 3; Brophy v. New England Mt. Sinai Hospital, Inc. see *supra*, note 1.

59. Superintendent of Belchertown State School v. Saikewicz, see *supra*, note 12.

60. In re Peter, see *supra*, note 32.

61. Millman v. First Federal Savings and Loan Ass'n., 198 So.2d 338 (Florida District Court of Appeal, 1967).

62. Brophy v. New England Mt. Sinai Hospital, Inc., see *supra*, note 1; Superintendent of Belchertown State School v. Saikewicz,, see *supra*, note 12; In re Guardianship of Estelle M. Browning, see *supra*, note 29; In re Spring, see *supra*, note 42.

63. In re Drabick, 200 Cal. App. 3rd 185, 245 Cal. Rptr. 840 (California Court of Appeal, 1988), *rev. den.* (July 28, 1988), *cert. den.* 109 S. Ct. 399 (1988); In re Guardianship of Hamlin, 102 Wash. 2d 810, 689 P.2d 1372 (Washington Supreme Court, 1984); Matter of Claire Conroy, see *supra*, note 8; Rasmussen v. Fleming, see *supra*, note 3.

64. In re Severns, 425 A.2d 156 (Delaware Court of Chancery, New Castle County, 1980); In re Guardianship of Hamlin, see *supra*, note 63.

65. 380 N.E.2d 134 (Massachusetts Appeals Court, Norfolk, 1978).

66. In re Conservatorship of Helga M. Wanglie (No. PX-91-283 Probate Court, Hennepin County, Minn., June 28, 1991).

67. In re Baby "K," 16F. 3rd 590, *petition for rehearing en banc denied*, No. 93-1899 (L) CA-93-68-A 28 March (4th Cir., 1940).

68. Florida Statutes, sec. 765.101 (1).

69. Florida Statutes, sec. 765.307 (5).

70. Dred Scott v. Sandford, 60 U.S. (19 Howard) 393 (1857).

71. Schecter Poultry Corporation v. U.S., 295 U.S. 495 (1935).

72. Severns v. Wilmington Medical Center, Inc., 421 A.2d 1334 (Delaware Supreme Court, 1980), where the Delaware Supreme Court stated: "We earnestly invite the prompt attention of the General Assembly with the hope that it will enact a comprehensive State policy governing these matters which are, in the words of Quinlan, of 'transcendent importance' "; In re Guardianship of Estelle M. Browning, see *supra*, note 29, where the District Court of Florida stated at 543 So.2d 270: "The legislature could clearly enact a more sophisticated remedy or create procedures based on interests in addition to the patient's constitutional right of privacy"; Satz v. Perlmutter, see *supra*, note 12, where the Florida Supreme Court said that the question raised by the refusal of life support by a competent, terminally ill patient "is not one which is well suited for resolution in an adversary judicial proceeding. It is the type which is more suitably addressed in the legislative forum."

73. Omnibus Budget Reconciliation Act 1990, Title IV, Public Law 101-508, section 4206; Amends several sections of 42 U.S. Code, in particular, sections 1395 cc (f) and 1396 a (w).

74. *Id.* at sec. 4206E.

References

American College of Physicians Ethics Committee. 1989. "American College of Physicians Ethics Manual, II." *Annals of Internal Medicine* 111:333.

Annas, G. J. 1991. "The Health Care Proxy and the Living Will." *New England Journal of Medicine* 324:1210–1213.

———. 1990. "Sounding Board: Nancy Cruzan and the Right to Die." *New England Journal of Medicine* 323:670–673.

———. 1988. "The Paradoxes of Organ Transplantation." *American Journal of Public Health* 78:621–622.

Annas, G. J., and Glantz, L. H. 1986. "The Right of Elderly Patients to Refuse Life-Sustaining Treatment." *Millbank Quarterly* 64:95–162.

Applebaum, P. S., and Grisso, T. 1988. "Assessing Patient's Capacities to Consent to Treatment." *New England Journal of Medicine* 319:1635–1638.

Beauchamp, T. L., and Childress, J. F. 1989. *Principles of Biomedical Ethics*. 3rd ed. New York: Oxford University Press.

Bedell, S. E., and Delbanco, T. L. 1984. "Choices about Cardiopulmonary Resuscitation in the Hospital: When Do Physicians Talk with Patients?" *New England Journal of Medicine* 310:1089–1093.

Bedell, S. E., Delbanco, T. L., Cook, E. F., and Epstein, F. H. 1983. "Survival after Cardiopulmonary Resuscitation in the Hospital." *New England Journal of Medicine* 309:569–576.

Bedell, S. E., Pelle, D., Maher, P. L., and Cleary, P. D. 1986. "Do-Not-Resuscitate Orders for Critically Ill Patients in the Hospital: How Are They Used and What Is Their Impact?" *Journal of the American Medical Association* 256:233–237.

Berger, A. S. 1993. *Dying and Death in Law and Medicine: A Forensic Primer for Health and Legal Professionals*. Westport, CT: Praeger.

Blackhall, L. J. 1987. "Must We Always Use CPR?" *New England Journal of Medicine* 317:1281–1285.

Callahan, D. 1991. "Medical Futility, Medical Necessity: The Problem-Without-a-Name."
    Hastings Center Report 21:30–35.
Cohen, Morris R. 1933. "The Basis of Contract." *Harvard Law Review* 46:553–592, at 586.
Colby, William H. 1990. "Missouri Stands Alone." *Hastings Center Report* 20:5–6.
Collin, F. F., Lombard, J. L., Moses, A. L., and Spitler, H. 1984. *Drafting the Durable Power
    of Attorney: A Systems Approach.* Lexington, SC: R.P.W. Publishing Co.
Council on Ethical and Judicial Affairs, American Medical Association. 1992. "Decisions
    near the End of Life." *Journal of the American Medical Association* 267:2229–2233.
———. 1991. "Guidelines for the Appropriate Use of Do-Not-Resuscitate Orders." *Journal
    of the American Medical Association* 265:1868–1871.
———. 1986. "Withholding or Withdrawing Life-Prolonging Medical Treatment." *Opinion*
    2.18.
Danis, M. Southerland, L. I., Garrett, J. M., Smith, J. L., Hielma, F., Pickard, C. G., Egner,
    D. M., and Patrick, D. L. 1991. "A Prospective Study of Advance Directives for
    Life-Sustaining Care." *New England Journal of Medicine* 324:882–888.
Dixon, J. L., and Smalley, M. G. 1981. "Jehovah's Witnesses: The Surgical/Ethical Chal-
    lenge." *Journal of the American Medical Association* 246:2471–2472.
Emanuel, L. L., and Emanuel, E. J. 1989. "The Medical Directive: A New Comprehensive
    Advance Care Document." *Journal of the American Medical Association* 261:3288–
    3293.
Faber-Langendoen, K. 1991. "Resuscitation of Patients with Metastatic Cancer." *Archives of
    Internal Medicine* 151:235–239.
Fried, T. R., Stein, M. D., O'Sullivan, P. S., Brock, D. W., and Novack, D. H. 1993.
    "Physician Attitudes and Practices Regarding Life-Sustaining Treatment and Eutha-
    nasia." *Archives of Internal Medicine* 153:722–728.
Hastings Center. 1987. *Guidelines on the Termination of Life-Sustaining Treatment and Care
    of the Dying.* New York.
Joint Commission on Accreditation of Healthcare Organizations. 1987. *Accreditation Man-
    ual for Hospitals.* Chicago.
Kutner, J. S., Ruark, J. E., and Raffin, T. A. 1991. "Defining Patient Competence for Medical
    Decision Making." *Chest* 100:1404–1409.
Lipton, H. L. 1986. "Do-Not-Resuscitate Orders in a Community Hospital." *Journal of the
    American Medical Association* 256:1164–1169.
Lo, B. 1991. "Unanswered Questions about DNR Orders." *Journal of the American Medical
    Association* 265:1874–1875.
McCartney, J. J. 1990. "The Right to Die: Perspectives from the Catholic and Jewish
    Traditions." In A. S. Berger and J. Berger, eds., *To Die or Not to Die? Cross-Disciplinary,
    Cultural, and Legal Perspectives on the Right to Choose Death,* pp.13–24. Westport, CT:
    Praeger.
Meisel, A. 1991. "Legal Myths about Terminating Life Support." *Archives of Internal Medicine*
    151:1497–1502.
Mill, John Stuart. 1961. "On Liberty." In *The Utilitarians: An Introduction to the Principles
    of Morals and Legislation. Jeremy Bentham. Utilitarianism* and *On Liberty. John Stuart
    Mill.* New York: Dolphin Books.
Mittelberger, J. A., Lo, B., Martin, D., and Uhlmann, R. F. 1993. "Impact of a Procedure-
    Specific Do Not Resuscitate Order Form on Documentation of Do Not Resuscitate
    Orders." *Archives of Internal Medicine* 153:228–232.

Orentlicher, D. 1990. "Advance Medical Directives." *Journal of the American Medical Association* 263:2365–2367.

President's Commission for the Study of Ethical Problems in Medicine and Biomedicine and Behavioral Research. 1983. *Deciding to Forgo Life-Sustaining Treatment.* Washington, D.C.: Government Printing Office.

———. 1982. *Making Health Care Decisions: A Report on the Ethical and Legal Implications of Informed Consent in the Patient-Practitioner Relationship.* Washington, D.C.: Government Printing Office.

"Questions of Law Live on after Father Helps Son Die." 1989. *New York Times.* 7 May, p. 26, col. 1.

Rie, M. A. 1991. "The Limits of a Wish." *Hastings Center Report* 21:24–27.

Ruark, E. R., Raffin, T. A., and the Stanford University Medical Center on Ethics. 1988. "Initiating and Withdrawing Life Support: Principles and Practice in Adult Medicine." *New England Journal of Medicine* 318:25–30.

Scully, T., and Scully, C. 1987. *Playing God: The New World of Medical Choices.* New York: Simon and Schuster.

"Teen Shunned Medication." 1994. *Miami Herald,* 21 August, p. 1, col. 1.

Truog, R. D., Brett, A. S., and Frader, J. 1992. "The Problem with Futility." *New England Journal of Medicine* 326:1560–1564.

Weir, R. F., and Gostin, L. 1990. "Decisions to Abate Life-Sustaining Treatment for Nonautonomous Patients: Ethical Standards and Legal Liability for Physicians after Cruzan." *Journal of the American Medical Association* 264:1846–1853.

Youngner, S. J. 1988. "Who Defines Futility?" *Journal of the American Medical Association* 260:2094–2095.

Zinber, J. M. 1989. "Decisions for the Dying: An Empiric Study of Physicians' Attitudes on Advance Directives." *Vermont Law Review* 13:445–491.

Table of Cases

Application of the President and Directors of Georgetown College, 172 n.21

Baby "K," 66
Barber v. Superior Court of California, 171 n.3, 172 n.32
Bartling v. Superior Court of California, 29, 171 n.3, 173 n.37
Bouvia v. Superior Court, 171 n.3
Brooks, In re, 18, 172 n.15
Brophy v. New England Mt. Sinai Hospital, Inc., 12, 27, 28, 51, 171 n.1
Browning, In re Guardianship of Estelle M., 172 n.29, 174 n.72

Cobbs v. Grant, 172 n.8
Conroy, Matter of Claire, 16, 172 n.8
Corbett v. D'Allessandro, 172 n.32
Cruzan v. Director, Missouri Department of Health, 12, 17, 25, 27, 51, 171 n.2
Cruzan v. Harmon, 21, 40, 171 n.2

Delio v. Westchester County Medical Center, 171 n.3
Dinnerstein, In re, 64, 173 n.65
Drabick, In re, 173 n.63
Dred Scott v. Sandford, 174 n.70
Eichner v. Dillon, 171 n.3

Erickson v. Delgard, 172 n.8

Farrell, In re, 173 n.54

Garger v. New Jersey, 8 n.1
Gray v. Romeo, 173 n.38
Griswold v. Connecticut, 16, 172 n.9

Hamlin, In re Guardianship of, 173 n.63
Hathaway v. Worcester City Hospital, 173 n.40

Jobes, In re, 29, 30, 172 n.32
John F. Kennedy Memorial Hospital, Inc. v. The Honorable Donald H. Bludworth, 171 n.3
John F. Kennedy Memorial Hospital v. Heston, 20, 172 n.17

Leach v. Shapiro, 171 n.3

McConnell v. Beverly Enterprises-Connecticut, Inc.,172 n.19
Meyer v. Nebraska, 173 n.54
Millman v. First Federal Savings and Loan Ass'n., 173 n.61

Natanson v. Kline, 171 n.4

New Mexico *ex. rel.* Smith v. Fort, 171 n.3

Osborne, In re, 172 n.22

Palm Springs General Hospital, Inc. v.
    Martinez, 172 n.8
Parham, Commissioner, Department of
    Human Resources of Georgia v. J. R.,
    173 n.55
People v. Pierson, 172 n.16
Peter, In re, 172 n.32
Pierce v. Society of Sisters, 173 n.54
Pratt v. Davis, 171 n.6

Quinlan, In re, 2, 17, 21, 31, 51, 171 n.3

Rasmussen v. Fleming, 171 n.3
Requena, In re, 173 n.36
Roe v. Wade, 16, 172 n.10
Satz v. Perlmutter, 172 n.12, 174 n.72

Schecter Poultry Corporation v. U.S.,
    174 n.71
Schloendorff v. Society of New York
    Hospital, 171 n.7
Severns, In re, 173 n.64
Severns v. Wilmington Medical Center,
    Inc., 174 n.72
Spring, In re, 173 n.42
Storar, In re, 171 n.3
Strachan v. John F. Kennedy Memorial
    Hospital, 8 n.2
Superintendent of Belchertown State
    School v. Saikewicz, 30, 172 n.12

Union Pacific Railway Co. v. Botsford,
    171 n.5

Wanglie, In re Conservatorship of Helen
    M., 65–66, 173 n.66
Wons v. Public Health Trust, 172 n.22

Index

Abortion, 17
Advance directives, 5, 6, 7, 14, 31, 45, 46, 50, 51, 53, 54, 56, 57, 58, 59, 67, 75–76, 78; disposition of, 50–51 (*see* Form 3.2.6); do-not-resuscitate order and, 37, 64; questions and answers about, (*see* Form 3.2.1); rationale for, 33; types of, 33–34; who decides if none, 51. *See also* Living wills
Advances, medical, 1, 3, 4; meanings of, 1–3
American Medical Association, 27, 64, 67, 69
Anesthesia, consent to, 16 (*see* Form 1.1.3)
Arigo, Benny, 60, 61
Artificial feeding. *See* Artificial nutrition and hydration
Artificial nutrition and hydration, 5, 22, 26–27, 30, 39; direction in living will concerning, 37 (*see* Form 2.3.4); living will statutes and, 36, 37
Autonomy, 11, 12, 13, 16, 17, 18, 21, 75; do-not-resuscitate orders and, 65, 66, 67, 69

Baby "K," 66
Bartling v. Superior Court, 29

Blood, refusal of, 18–19; by Jehovah's Witnesses (*see* Form 1.1.4); by others (*see* Form 1.1.5)
Brooks, In re, 18
Brophy, Patricia, 11, 12, 28
Brophy, Paul, 11, 12, 30, 53
Brophy v. New England Mt. Sinai Hospital, 12, 17, 20, 25, 27, 28, 29, 30, 51
Brother Fox, 21, 40

Cardiopulmonary resuscitation, 3, 5, 67, 68, 69; code, chemical, 71; code, limited, 71; code, slow, 71; "code blue," 58, 63; "code pink," 59, 63; consent implied, 63; discussions with patients, 67–68; "no code," 58, 59, 63; oral consent to refuse, 70; progress notes, and, 70, 72; questions and answers about, 67 (*see* Form 5.1.1); refusal of by patient, 67 (*see* Form 5.1.2); refusal of by proxy or surrogate, 67, 70 (*see* Forms 1.3.4, 5.1.2); survival rate, 68; withholding, 63–73 *passim*. *See also* Do-not-resuscitate order
Civil War, 75
Clear and convincing evidence, 22, 39, 40, 41, 53, 58

Competence, 43, 44, 45, 47, 50, 52, 53,
    54, 60, 61. *See also* Patients, decision-
    making capacity in; Right to refuse
    life-sustaining treatment
Conroy, Matter of Claire, 16
Consent. *See* Informed consent
Courts, 1, 2, 15, 31, 58; do-not-resusci-
    tate orders and, 71–72; functions, 75;
    futility question and, 65–66, 71–72;
    guardianship proceedings and, 24;
    pregnancy and termination of life-sus-
    taining treatment by surrogate, 48 57;
    termination of life-sustaining treat-
    ment and approval of, 30–31
Cruzan, Nancy, 12, 21, 39, 41, 45, 53
*Cruzan v. Director, Missouri Department
    of Health*, 12, 17, 25, 27, 31, 36, 40,
    41, 44, 45, 51, 53, 57, 65
Cruzan v. Harmon, 12, 21, 40

Decision making. *See* Patients; Proxy;
    Surrogates
Decision-making capacity. *See* Patients
Department of Health and Rehabilitative
    Services, 60
Dinnerstein, In re, 64
Do-not-resuscitate order, 1, 3–4, 5, 6, 7,
    58, 59, 63–65, 67, 68; autonomy
    and, 65, 66, 69; conflict over, 69; con-
    sent to by patient, proxy, or surrogate,
    68, 69, 71, 72 (*see* Forms 5.1.3, 5.2.1,
    5.2.2); effect of, 63, 68, 72; emotion-
    laden problem, 70; form of order, 68,
    70 (*see* Form 5.1.4); not preclude
    other care, 70; oral, 72–73; patient
    participation in, 71; progress notes,
    70, 72 (*see* Form 5.2.1.2); questions
    and answers about, 67 (*see* Form
    5.1.1); refusal of CPR and emotion-
    laden problem, 70; revocation, 71; sus-
    pension, 71; unilateral issuance,
    63–64, 66, 69, 71–72; written, 70,
    72. *See also* Prehospital do-not-resusci-
    tate order
Dred Scott v. Sandford, 75
Durable power of attorney for health
    care, 7, 48–50 *passim*, 52, 53, 56, 75;

appointment of attorney-in-fact with
    broad powers (*see* Form 3.2.5.1); ap-
    pointment of attorney-in-fact for
    health care (*see* Form 3.2.5); copy of,
    50; health care surrogate designation
    compared, 49; incompetency of prin-
    cipal, determination of, 50, 52 (*see*
    Forms 3.2.5.2, 3.2.5.3); incompe-
    tency of principal, effect, 50; notariza-
    tion, 48; restrictions on consent by
    attorney-in-fact, 49; signing of, 48,
    52; "springing," 50; statutory differ-
    ences, 49; witnesses to, 48

Emanuel, Ezekiel, 37
Emanuel, Linda, 37
Emergency Medical Treatment and
    Woman in Active Labor Act, 66
End-of-life matters, 1, 2, 3; forms and, 6;
    hospital policies and, 8
Euthanasia, 27–28, 35
Extraordinary treatment. *See* Right to re-
    fuse life-sustaining treatment

Fairfax Hospital, 66
Forms, medicolegal, 3; defined, 6; impor-
    tance of, 6
Friend, close, 15, 31, 45, 52; affidavit by,
    52 (*see* Form 3.3.2)
Futility, 5, 60, 64, 66–68, 70, 72; adjudi-
    cation of question of, 65–66, 71–72;
    illustrations of, 72; physiological, 64,
    65; value-laden concept, 65

Griswold v. Connecticut, 16, 17
Guardian, legal, 15, 24, 31, 43, 46–47,
    51; consent to do-not-resuscitate or-
    der, 68 (*see* Form 5.1.3); decision to
    forgo life-sustaining treatment, 55–56
    (*see* Form 4.1.1); refusal of cardiopul-
    monary resuscitation, 67 (*see* Form
    5.1.2); refusal of treatment and re-
    lease, 24 (*see* Form 1.3.4)

Health care surrogate designation, 47,
    49, 50, 52, 53, 56, 75; advisory for pa-
    tients (*see* Form 3.2.3); alternate surro-

gate, 47; annulment of marriage, effect of, 48; authority, scope, 47–48; authority, when begins, 47; competence of principal, 47; copies of designation, 47, 50; designation of, 47 (*see* Forms 3.2.4, 3.2.4.1, 3.2.4.2); designation, signing of, 47, 52; divorce, effect of, 48; health care surrogate designation and living will compared, 47; pregnancy and, 48; restrictions on consent by, 48, 52; withholding life-sustaining procedures, instructions, 47 (*see* Form 3.2.4.1); witnesses to, 47, 52

Health professionals. *See* Hospitals; Nurses; Physicians

Health providers. *See* Hospitals; Nurses; Physicians

Hennepin County Medical Center, 65

Hippocrates, 28

Homicide, 12, 26, 27, 35

Hospitals: abandonment of patient and, 28; advance directives, 36, 51, 52 (*see* Form 3.3.1 for policy); cardiopulmonary resuscitation, emotion-laden problem and, 70 (*see* Form 5.2.1.1); cardiopulmonary resuscitation, refusal of by patient, 67 (*see* Form 5.1.2); cardiopulmonary resuscitation, refusal of by proxy or surrogate, 67, 70 (*see* Forms 1.3.4, 5.1.2); conflict between patients' rights and policies, 28, 30, 35; court proceedings and, 15, 31; decision-making capacity, 23–24, 55, 71; disputes with patients, 2; do-not-resuscitate orders and, 3–4, 67, 68, 71 (*see* Form 5.1.1 for questions and answers for patients, Form 5.1.2 for patient refusal of CPR, and Form 5.1.3 for patient, proxy, or surrogate consent to DNR order); do-not-resuscitate orders, policies on, 69 (*see* Forms 5.2.1 and 5.2.2); emotion-laden problems, 59–60, 70 (*see* Forms 4.2.3.1, 5.2.1.1); false imprisonment and, 29; futility and, 65; guardianship proceedings, 24, 71 (*see* Forms 1.3.1.1,

5.2.1.3); informed consent and, 14–15 (*see* Form 1.1.1 for policy); Jehovah's Witnesses and, 18–19; law and, 3–4; liability, immunity from, 34; living will documentation, 36, 52; living will notification, 35–36, 38; living will statutes and, 35, 46; medicolegal forms and, 3; minor's decision, 61 (*see* Form 4.2.3.3); minor's participation in decisions, 61 (*see* Form 4.2.3.2); mission and right to refuse treatment, 28, 30, 35; Patient Self-Determination Act, and, 76, 77, 78 (*see* Forms 6.1.1 and 6.1.2 for written information required for patients, Form 6.1.4 for checklist for hospital representative, and Form 6.2.1 for policy); pediatric patients and emotion-laden problem, 59–60 (*see* Form 4.2.3.1 for alternative clause in withholding or withdrawing life-sustaining treatment policy); philosophy of, 28, 30; policies and, 7–8, 23–25, 28–29, 35, 52; pregnancy and refusal of life-sustaining treatment, and, 25, 57 (*see* Form 1.3.1.2 for optional clause); refusal of treatment and, 23–25 (*see* Form 1.3.1 for policy); refusal of treatment by guardian, 24 (*see* Form 1.3.4); refusal of treatment by patient, 23, 67 (*see* Form 1.2.1); refusal of treatment by proxy, 24, 67, 70 (*see* Form 1.3.4); refusal of treatment by surrogate, 24, 67, 70 (*see* Form 1.3.4); religious beliefs and, 18; social services department, 24; surrogate, challenge of, 31–32; termination of life support and court approval, 30–31; transfer of patient, 29–30, 35, 58; when cannot find surrogate or proxy, 15; withholding or withdrawing life-sustaining treatment from terminally ill adults, 56–58 *passim*, 78 (*see* Form 4.2.1 for policy); withholding or withdrawing life-sustaining treatment from terminally ill pediatric patients, 58–59 (*see* Form 4.2.2 for policy)

Informed consent, 6, 7, 12, 13–14, 16, 18,
    19, 23, 43, 44, 60, 69, 70; capacity to
    give, 15, 23, 24; emergency and, 14;
    forms of, 15; hospital policy (*see* Form
    1.1.1); living will and, 36–37; special
    consent form (*see* Form 1.1.2)

Jackson Memorial Hospital, 60
Jehovah's Witnesses, 18, 20, 25; refusal
    of blood transfusion form, 18 (*see*
    Form 1.1.4). *See also* Religious beliefs
Jobes, In re, 29, 30
*John F. Kennedy Memorial Hospital v.
    Heston*, 20
Joint Commission on Accreditation of
    Healthcare Organizations, 69
Judges, 1, 2

Law, common, 1, 2, 25, 39, 50; role of,
    2; written, 1, 2
Lawmakers, 1, 2
Lawyers, 3
Legislators, 2
Liberty interest, 12, 17, 18, 65
Life, preservation of, 12, 21–22
Life-sustaining treatment, 4, 16, 17, 19–
    22, 27, 53–54, 57, 67, 75; do-not-re-
    suscitate order and, 64; withdrawing,
    1, 5, 6, 7, 11, 18, 26, 30, 48, 49, 55–
    61 *passim*; withholding, 1, 5, 6, 7, 11,
    18, 30, 48, 49, 55–61 *passim*. *See also*
    Artificial nutrition and hydration;
    Right to refuse life-sustaining treat-
    ment
Living wills, 1, 5, 27, 33, 39, 41, 45, 46,
    49, 50, 52, 53, 75; additional direc-
    tions, 37 (*see* Form 2.3.4); artificial
    feeding and, 36; cardiopulmonary re-
    suscitation and, 68; copies of, 50, 51;
    decision-making capacity and, 36–37;
    designation of surrogate, 46 (*see* Form
    3.2.2); direction concerning artificial
    feeding, 37 (*see* Form 2.3.4); direction
    concerning pain control, 37; do-not-
    resuscitate order and, 37, 64, 69;
    euthanasia and, 35; executed in other
    states, 35; form, 35, 36, 38 (*see* Forms
    2.3.2, 2.3.3); health care surrogate desig-
    nation compared, 47; homicide and,
    35; life insurance and, 35; notarization
    of, 38; notification to health care facility
    or physician, 35–36, 38; Patient Self-
    Determination Act, 1, 5, 6, 7, 36, 67,
    75–78 *passim*; pregnancy and, 37–38
    (*see* Forms 2.36, 2.3.7); questions and
    answers about, 36 (*see* Form 2.3.1);
    revocation of, 38, 52 (*see* Form 2.3.8);
    signing of, 38; specification of proce-
    dures, 37; statutes, 33–35, 36, 37, 38,
    40, 46, 57, 58, 60; suicide and, 35; sur-
    rogate, designation of, 46 (*see* Form
    3.2.2); terminal condition and, 34, 36,
    46, 56; witnesses to, 38; who may
    make, 34. *See also* Advance directives
Long-term care facilities. *See* Nursing
    homes

Medical profession, 2; do-not-resuscitate
    order and, 64, 66, 67; ethics, 28; state
    and integrity of, 21
Meisel, Alan, 25
Minor children, 5, 7, 15, 19, 24, 40;
    emotion-laden problem, 59–60, 70;
    mature minors, 60–61; religious be-
    liefs and, 19; state interest and, 19,
    20–21; terminal illness, certification
    of, 59 (*see* Form 4.2.3); termination
    of treatment and emotion-laden prob-
    lem, 59–60, 70; withholding or with-
    drawing life-sustaining procedures
    from terminally ill pediatric patients,
    58–59 (*see* Form 4.2.2 for hospital
    policy). *See also* Proxy
Missouri Compromise, 75
Mt. Vernon State Hospital, 39

National Recovery Act, 75
New England Mt. Sinai Hospital, 11,
    28, 30
Nurses: cardiopulmonary resuscitation,
    progress notes and, 70; forms and, 6;
    hospital policies and, 7, 8; Jehovah's
    Witnesses and, 18–19; moral beliefs
    and, 29; refusal of treatment and, 23

Nursing homes, 7, 8, 30, 46; policies and right to refuse treatment, 28–29

O'Connor, Sandra Day, 45
Omnibus Budget Reconciliation Act, 75

Patients: advance directives and, 33; adult, 5, 7, 14, 15, 17, 20, 22, 23, 25, 26, 29, 30; anesthesia, consent to, 16 (*see* Form 1.1.3); autonomy, 11, 66; cardiopulmonary resuscitation, discussions with physicians, 67–68, 69; cardiopulmonary resuscitation, refusal of, 67, 69 (*see* Forms 1.2.1, 5.1.2); conflict between rights and hospital policies, 28, 29, 35; decision-making capacity, 5, 7, 15, 18, 23, 24, 33, 36–37, 38, 41, 43, 47, 48, 51, 52, 55, 57, 67, 68, 70, 71; disputes with health providers, 2; do-not-resuscitate orders, and, 63, 64, 66, 67 65, 66, 68, 69 (*see* Form 5.1.2 for refusal of CPR and Form 5.1.3 for consent to DNR order); informed consent (*see* Informed consent); not terminally ill, 23; pediatric, 5, 7, 15, 24, 58–61; physician-patient relationship, 26, 28; policies of health care facilities and, 28–29; pregnancy and, 25, 48; refusal of treatment, 23, 67 (*see* Form 1.2.1); terminally ill, 7, 16, 25, 46, 54, 55, 56, 67, 68; termination of life support and court approval, 30–31; transfer of, 29–30, 35. *See also* Autonomy; Informed consent; Liberty interest; Life-sustaining treatment; Privacy right; Religious beliefs; Right to refuse life-sustaining treatment
Patient Self-Determination Act, 1, 5, 6, 7, 36, 67, 75–78 *passim*
Physicians: advance directives and, 33, 46, 77 (*see* Form 6. 1.3 for informing patients); cardiopulmonary resuscitation, discussions with patient, proxy, surrogate, 67–68, 70; cardiopulmonary resuscitation, emotional problem and, 70; cardiopulmonary resuscita-

tion, progress notes and, 70 (*see* Form 5.2.1.2); cardiopulmonary resuscitation, refusal of, 67, 69, 70 (*see* Forms 1.2.1, 1.3.4, 5.1.2); certification of decision-making capacity, 54, 56, 57 (*see* Form 3.4.1); certification of terminal condition, 54, 56, 59 (*see* Form 3.4.1 for adult patients, Form 4.2.3 for pediatric patients); concerns, 11–12; conflicts between patients' rights and moral beliefs, 28, 29, 35; decision-making capacity and, 23–24, 43, 44, 54, 55, 70 (*see also* Patients); disputes with patients, 2, 11, 16; do-not-resuscitate orders and, 3–4, 63–64, 65, 66, 67, 68, 69, 70 (*see* Form 5.1.1 for questions and answers for patients, Form 5.1.2 for patient refusal of CPR, Form 5.1.3 for consent by patient, proxy, or surrogate to DNR order, and Form 5.1.4 for DNR order); emotion-laden problems, 59–60, 70; forms and, 6; futility and, 63–65; hospital policies and, 7, 8; informed consent and, 14; Jehovah's Witnesses and, 18–19; law and, 3–4; liability, immunity from, 34, 46, 78; living wills and, 34, 35, 36, 38, 39, 46; medicolegal forms and, 3; moral beliefs and, 12, 28, 29, 70–71, 72; not forced to provide treatment, 29, 70–71; Patient Self-Determination Act and, 76, 77, 78; pediatric patients and emotion-laden problem, 59–60; physician-patient relationship, 26, 28; progress notes, 70, 72 (*see* Form 5.2.1.2); proxy and, 24; refusal of treatment and, 23; refusal of treatment by guardian, 24 (*see* Form 1.3.4); refusal of treatment by patient, 23, 67 (see Form 1.2.1); refusal of treatment by proxy, 24, 67 (*see* Form 1.3.4); religious beliefs and, 18; surrogates and, 24, 54; terminal illness and, 34, 54, 55–56, 59; transfer of patient, 29–30, 35, 58, 71; withdrawal from case, 70; withholding or withdrawing life-sus-

taining treatment from adult terminally ill patients, 11–12, 57–58
Policies, hospital, 3, 7–8, 76; adult terminally ill patients, withholding or withdrawing life-sustaining treatment
from, 56–58 *passim*, 78 (*see* Form
4.2.1); advance directives and, 36, 51,
52, 76, 78 (*see* Forms 3.3.1, 6.2.1);
cardiopulmonary resuscitation, emotional problem and, 70 (*see* Form
5.2.1.1); do-not-resuscitate orders, 69
(see Forms 5.2.1, 5.2.2); guardianship
proceedings, 24, 71 (see Forms
1.3.1.1, 5.2.1.3); informed consent
and, 14 (*see* Form 1.1.1); minor's decision, acceptance of, 61 (*see* Form
4.2.3.3); minor's participation in decisions, 61 (*see* Form 4.2.3.2); oral consent to CPR, 70 (*see* Form 5.2.1.1);
Patient Self Determination Act and,
76, 77, 78 (*see* Form 6. 2.1); pediatric
patients and emotion-laden problems,
59–60, 70 (*see* Form 4.2.3.1 for alternative clause in withholding or withdrawing life-sustaining treatment
policy); pediatric terminally ill patients, withholding or withdrawing
life-sustaining treatment from, 58–59
(*see* Form 4.2.2); pregnancy and refusal of life-sustaining treatment, 25
(*see* Form 1.3.1.2 for optional clause);
proxy's oral consent to CPR, 70 (*see*
Form 5.2.1.1); refusal of treatment
and, 23 (*see* Form 1.3.1); surrogate's
oral consent to CPR, 70 (*see* Form
5.2.1.1); withholding or withdrawing
life-sustaining treatment from terminally ill adults, 56–58 *passim* (*see*
Form 4.2.1); withholding or withdrawing life-sustaining treatment
from terminally ill pediatric patients,
58–59 (*see* Form 4.2.2)
Power of attorney, 48–49, 50. *See also*
Durable power of attorney for health
care
Pregnancy, 25, 37–38, 57

Prehospital do-not-rescuscitate order, 5,
73–74 (*see* Form 5.3.1). *See also* Do-
not-resuscitate order
President's Commission for the Study of
Ethical Problems in Medicine and
Biomedicine and Behavioral Research,
26, 40
Privacy right, 12, 16–17, 18, 65
Procedures, hospital. *See* Policies, hospital
Proxy: authority, when begins, 52; best
interest test, 53–54, 55, 58; cardiopulmonary resuscitation, refusal of, 67,
70 (*see* Forms 1.3.4, 5.1.2); consent to
do-not-resuscitate order, 68 (*see* Form
5.1.3); decision forgoing life-sustaining treatment, 55–56, 57, 58 (*see*
Form 4.1.1 and Form 4.2.4 for terminally ill pediatric patient); decision
making, 54, 55; decisions, scope of,
52–53; do-not-resuscitate orders and,
63–64, 65; informed consent and, 14,
15; life-sustaining treatment, decision
to forgo, 55–56, 57, 58 (*see* Form
4.1.1 and Form 4.2.4 for terminally
ill pediatric patient); minors, consent
for, 15, 60, 61 (*see* Forms 1.1.2,
4.2.4) notification to, 24, 52, 56 (*see*
Form 1.3.3); objective test, 53; order
of priority, 14–15, 31, 51; pediatric
patients and, 59–50; procedure for selection if no advance directive, 51; refusal of cardiopulmonary
resuscitation, 67, 70 (*see* Forms 1.3.4,
5.1.2); refusal of treatment and release, 24, 53 (*see* Form 1.3.4); refusal
of treatment by, 23; restriction on
consent by, 15; selection of, 14–15,
52; standards for decision making, 23,
24, 53; subjective standard, 23, 24,
53, 54, 55; substituted judgment test,
23, 52, 54, 55, 56, 58, 61; withdrawing life-sustaining treatment, 55, 56,
57, 58–59, 65; withholding life-sustaining treatment, 55, 56, 57, 58–59,
61, 65

Quinlan, In re, 2, 17, 18, 21, 26, 31, 51,
53, 65, 75
Quinlan, Karen Ann, 2, 11, 33

Refusal of life-sustaining treatment, 16,
60, 78; guardian, 24 (*see* Form 1.3.4);
hospital policy, 23 (*see* Form 1.3.1);
patient, 23, 67 (*see* Form 1.2.1);
proxy, 24, 67 (*see* Form 1.3.4); surrogate, 24, 67 (*see* Form 1.3.4). *See also*
Life-sustaining treatment; Patients;
Proxy; Right to refuse life-sustaining
treatment; Surrogate
Rehnquist, William, 17
Religious beliefs, 17; minor children and,
20–21
Requena, In re, 29
Right to die, 17, 18
Right to refuse life-sustaining treatment:
artificial nutrition and hydration and,
27, 36; autonomy and, 16, 22; competence and, 12, 22, 33, 44, 60–61; decision-making capacity and, 43 (*see also*
Patients); distinction between "extraordinary" and "ordinary," and, 25–
26; distinction between withholding
and withdrawing treatment, 26; emergency situation and, 24; euthanasia
and, 27; "extraordinary" treatment
and, 26; form for refusal by patient
(*see* Form 1.2.1); incompetence and,
44–45; informed consent and, 16, 22;
liberty interest and, 17, 22; limitation
of to terminally ill, 25; loss of, 45, 47;
policies of health care facilities and,
28–29; pregnancy and, 25, 57; preservation of life and, 21–22; privacy
right and, 17, 22; proxy by, 24; quality of life and, 44; religious beliefs
and, 18–19, 22; state interests and,
19–22; surrogate by, 24; treatment already started and, 26; withholding
and withdrawing treatment and, 26.
See also Life-sustaining treatment
Roe v. Wade, 16, 17

Self-determination. *See* Autonomy

State interests, 19–22, 40
Suicide, 20; living wills and, 35; prevention of, 20; state interest and, 20
*Superintendent of Belchertown State School
v. Saikewicz*, 30
Surrogates, 1, 5, 6, 7, 30, 38, 45; annulment of marriage, effect of, 46, 48;
best interest test, 53–54, 55; cardiopulmonary resuscitation, refusal of,
67, 70 (*see* Forms 1.3.4, 5.1.2); consent to do-not-resuscitate order, 68
(*see* Form 5.1.3); decision forgoing
life-sustaining treatment, 55–56, 57
(*see* Forms 4.1.1, 4.1.1.1); decision
making, 1, 14, 45, 54; decisions, challenge of, 31–32, 52; decisions, scope
of, 52–53, 55; designation of, 45, 46,
46 (*see* Forms 3.2.2, 3.2.3); divorce,
effect of, 46, 48; do-not-resuscitate orders and, 63–64, 65; family as, 40–
41, 45, 51; health care surrogate
designation, 47 (*see also* Health care
surrogate designation); informed consent and, 14, 15; judicial review of decisions, 31–32, 52; life-sustaining
treatment, decision to forgo, 55–56,
57 (*see* Forms 4.1.1, 4.1.1.1); living
will designation of, 46 (*see* Form
3.2.2); mechanisms for decision making, 45–50 *passim*; no power to consent to certain procedures, 15;
notification to, 24, 52, 56 (*see* Form
1.3.2); objective test, 53; pregnant patient's delegation or nondelegation of
authority, 38, 57 (*see* Form 2.3.7); refusal of cardiopulmonary resuscitation, 67, 70 (*see* Forms 1.3.4, 5.1.2);
refusal of treatment and release by,
24, 53 (*see* Form 1.3.4); restrictions
on consent by, 48, 52; restrictions on
who can serve as, 47; revocation of
designation, 46; spouse as, 46; standards for decision making, 23, 24, 53;
subjective standard, 23, 24, 53, 54;
substituted judgment test, 23, 53, 54,
55, 56; withdrawing life-sustaining
treatment, 55, 56, 65; withholding

life-sustaining treatment, 55, 56, 65.
    See also Health care surrogate
Surrogate decision making. *See* Surrogates

Technology, medical, 1, 2
Terminally ill. *See* Living wills; Patients;
    Physicians
Termination of treatment. *See* Do-not-re-
    suscitate order; Life-sustaining treatment

U. S. Department of Health and Human
    Services, 76

Wanglie, Helen, 65–66
Wanglie, Oliver, 65–66
Withdrawing life-sustaining treatment.
    See Hospitals; Life-sustaining treat-
    ment; Policies, hospital; Proxy; Right
    to refuse life-sustaining treatment; Sur-
    rogate
Withholding life-sustaining treatment.
    See Hospitals; Life-sustaining treat-
    ment; Policies, hospital; Proxy; Right
    to refuse life-sustaining treatment; Sur-
    rogate

ABOUT THE AUTHOR

ARTHUR S. BERGER is the Director of the International Institute for the Study of Death. Listed in *Who's Who in the World* and *Who's Who in the South and Southwest*, he is the author of more than thirty papers and several books on thanatology including *Dying and Death in Law and Medicine* (Praeger, 1992), *To Die or Not to Die* (Praeger, 1990), and *Perspectives on Death and Dying* (1989).

ISBN 0-275-94620-7

90000>

HARDCOVER BAR CODE